Angela Kubbs. 1992.

122-95

CW00557953

A Manual of
Labour Ward Practice

A Manual of
Labour Ward Practice

J. Malcolm Pearce FRCS MRCOG
Senior Lecturer

and

Shirley A. Steel MB MRCOG
Research Registrar

The Fetal Welfare Laboratory
Department of Obstetrics and Gynaecology
St George's Hospital Medical School
London, UK

A Wiley Medical Publication

JOHN WILEY & SONS
Chichester · New York · Brisbane · Toronto · Singapore

Copyright © 1987 by John Wiley & Sons Ltd.

All rights reserved.

No part of this book may be reproduced by any means, or transmitted, or translated into a machine language without the written permission of the publisher

Library of Congress Cataloging-in-Publication Data:

Pearce, J. Malcolm (John Malcolm)
  A manual of labour ward practice.

  (A Wiley medical publication)
  Bibliography: p.
  Includes index.
  1. Labor (Obstetrics) 2. Labor, Complicated.
3. Obstetrical nursing. I. Steel, Shirley.
II. Title. III. Series.
RG651.P43 1987   618.4   87-8107

ISBN 0 471 91195 X

British Library Cataloguing in Publication Data:

Pearce, J. Malcolm
  A manual of labour ward practice.
  1. Gynecologic nursing
  2. Obstetrical nursing
  I. Title II. Steel, Shirley
  610.73'678   RG105

ISBN 0 471 91195 X

Printed and bound in Great Britain
by Biddles Ltd., Guildford.

Contents

Preface

The purpose of this book is to provide a comprehensive and practical guide to the management of women in labour for all health workers involved in their care.

Part I is an introduction to the labour ward with suggested guidelines for equipment and personnel; Part II covers various aspects of normal labour and delivery. These two sections could be read at leisure, whilst Part III should provide on-the-spot advice in complicated situations.

The suggestions for management obviously largely reflect the authors' personal viewpoints, but we hope that our approach is seen to be direct and logical, and that this book will prove to be useful to midwives and medical staff who hope to ensure that labour is not only a momentous and enjoyable experience, but also a safe one.

J. M. PEARCE
S. A. STEEL

Acknowledgements

The authors would like to thank Mrs Jill Edwards for her patience in typing this book, the St George's Hospital Medical School audiovisual department for their assistance with all the photographs, and Dr N. McIntosh, Consultant Paediatrician at St George's Hospital, for his advice as to the content of Chapter 6 concerning neonatal resuscitation. We would also like to express our thanks to all the consultants, medical and midwifery staff who contributed with their comments and suggestions to the labour ward protocol currently in use on the labour ward at St George's Hospital and which formed the basis for this book.

J. M. PEARCE
S. A. STEEL

Introduction

The Labour Ward

Design, planning and facilities

Labour ward staff

Expectations of the pregnant woman

The delivery

DESIGN, PLANNING AND FACILITIES

The ideal labour ward is a purpose-built area with adequate facilities to ensure the safety of the woman in labour, her fetus and the neonate. At the same time it should provide an environment for delivery which simulates the home as much as possible as the vast majority of women will experience an uncomplicated and straightforward pregnancy and delivery.

The optimum number of delivery rooms will depend upon the expected number of deliveries (see Table 1). Ideally there should be a single room available to each woman for the duration of her labour. Formerly, women were transferred to a second stage room when the cervix was fully dilated, having spent the first stage in a large room with other women in labour. However, this practice was not ideal, for several reasons. The first stage room allows minimal privacy for the woman and her partner, and her anxiety and apprehension may be compounded by witnessing other women's reactions to labour. It is also unreasonable to move women at a time when they are experiencing maximal discomfort and a strong urge to push.

Each labour ward should contain at least one larger delivery room that can accommodate the additional personnel and technology required for the delivery of a breech or multiple pregnancy. In addition facilities should be available for intensive nursing. Ideally this should be within the confines of the labour ward and the nursing should be carried out by midwives. Every labour ward should be capable of managing very ill patients and only in situations where ventilation or dialysis, for instance, is required should pregnant or puerperal women be moved to other wards.

There should ideally be a sufficient number of fetal heart rate monitors to allow every patient in labour to be monitored at any one time if necessary (see Table 1). Provision should be made for the use of telemetry (see Figure 2.3) which allows full mobility of the women whilst recording the fetal heart rate and uterine contractions.

Table 1   Facilities for the labour ward

One delivery room	per 300 deliveries
One operating theatre (*en suite*)	per 1500–2000 deliveries
One CTG machine	per 500 deliveries
One pH machine	per labour ward
One resuscitaire	per 300 deliveries

This has the obvious attraction of providing no limitation to movement whilst still providing information regarding fetal well-being.

Abnormal fetal heart rate patterns should be backed up by fetal scalp pH to detect intrapartum asphyxia, since basing decisions on heart rate pattern alone increases the Caesarean section rate without improving perinatal outcome. At least two sets of equipment for scalp sampling and one blood gas machine should therefore be available on every labour ward.

There must be instant access to an operating theatre and a dedicated *en suite* operating theatre should be provided for every 1500–2000 deliveries (see Table 1).

A small portable real-time ultrasound machine with on-screen measuring facilities is a useful addition to each labour ward and is vital in centres attached to regional neonatal units. It is used for:

1. Confirming fetal viability or death.
2. Localizing the placenta in cases of antepartum haemorrhage prior to speculum examination (see Chapter 12).
3. Estimating fetal weight in unbooked patients, those in preterm labour (see Chapter 9) and in those with an undiagnosed breech (see Chapter 19).
4. Confirming fetal presentation.
5. Excluding major fetal malformations prior to Caesarean section for preterm infants.

A reasonable variety of instruments for operative vaginal delivery should be available, including Andersons, Wrigleys and Kjellands forceps and a Ventouse or vacuum extractor. Destructive instruments are unnecessary.

LABOUR WARD STAFF

The smooth and efficient running of a labour ward depends upon the numbers of staff available, their training, experience and attitudes. The optimum number of staff are outlined in Table 2.

Medical and midwifery staff should have a relaxed and flexible attitude to the management of normal labour. Good communication, between the staff and patients, and between colleagues is absolutely essential, particularly at the times of change-over of shifts.

Table 2   Staff

Midwifery

One midwife per patient.
One senior labour ward sister per labour ward.

Obstetric

One senior house officer per 3000 deliveries (with sole duties on labour ward).
One registrar per labour ward (with sole duties if >3500 deliveries).
Consultant cover 24 hours per day.

Anaesthetic

One registrar (with sole duties if >3500 deliveries).
Consultant cover 24 hours per day.

In an ideal situation, a midwife's duties should be flexible enough to allow her to stay with a particular woman for the duration of her labour. Standards of care will be improved by regular supervision and input from a senior level of obstetric, anaesthetic, paediatric and midwifery staff. Regular ward rounds should occur throughout the day with an emphasis upon continuity of care. Opportunities should exist for continuing in-training education at all levels.

Occasionally, in urgent situations the need for hasty action means that the woman and her partner are given only a brief explanation of the situation and the decisions that need to be made. As soon as is feasible after the event a full explanation and discussion of the sequence of events should take place.

EXPECTATIONS OF THE PREGNANT WOMAN

All pregnant women expect to leave the labour ward with a live, healthy baby. This is the ideal which all labour ward staff should strive to achieve. The health and safety of both mother and baby is the first priority in antenatal and intrapartum care.

Fortunately women now have ample opportunity to become well-informed about pregnancy, with the abundance of literature available, and the provision of antenatal and/or parentcraft classes in most hospitals. There should be the opportunity for an accurate explanation and discussion whenever the woman has any anxieties or queries, or whenever complications arise, during pregnancy or labour.

Many women have express wishes concerning the manner in which their labour and delivery should be conducted. They may feel that they need to put these views on paper as a birth plan. The points raised in such a birth plan should be fully discussed before labour. If midwifery and medical staff feel that by following the plan the woman or her baby may be put at unnecessary risk, these risks should be appreciated by the woman. Otherwise, every attempt should be made to fulfil her wishes.

Verbal consent should be obtained for all procedures to which the woman may be subjected during labour, and written consent is required should she request epidural analgesia or require Caesarean section.

THE DELIVERY

Throughout her labour the woman should ideally be accompanied by her attendant midwife and a companion of her choice. She should be made as comfortable as possible at all stages of her labour. She may choose to lie on the delivery bed when she should be sitting up or on one side, or she may wish to use a bean bag or rocking chair. The presence, moral support and companionship of her partner, friend or relative is important and participation should be encouraged.

The most comfortable and effective position for delivery should be sought after discussion between the woman and her midwife. Provided her midwife feels that she is able to conduct the delivery safely, a flexible attitude to maternal wishes should be maintained. A birthing chair may be available for the woman's use if she wishes.

To maintain privacy as far as possible every person should knock and wait to be told to come in before entering the delivery room. When a person unknown to the woman enters her delivery room they should introduce themselves and explain their role. If the woman expresses a desire not to be accompanied by medical or midwifery students, then these wishes should be upheld.

After delivery, the baby should be allowed to stay with its mother as much as possible, both on the labour ward and on the postnatal ward. Women who wish to breast feed should be allowed to put their baby to the breast as soon after delivery as is practical.

PART I

NORMAL LABOUR AND DELIVERY

Chapter 1

Normal Labour and Delivery

1.1 ADMISSION CRITERIA

Women who attend the labour ward will fall into one of two groups:

1. Those who suspect that they are in spontaneous normal labour.
2. Those with specific symptoms or problems requiring assessment.

Admission is usually advised for:

1. Regular painful contractions. When the frequency exceeds one contraction in 10

min in a primigravida or one in 20 min in a multigravida, admission is usually advised.

2.   Spontaneous rupture of membranes.

Any patient who telephones the labour ward expressing concern must be advised to attend for assessment. Such complaints may be of reduced fetal movements, abdominal pain or vaginal bleeding. In the case of the latter, the amount and nature of the bleeding should be ascertained. If there is any doubt, or bleeding is profuse, then the obstetric flying squad should be sent to the woman's home (see Chapter 34).

1.2   ADMISSION PROCEDURE

Each woman should ideally be admitted by the midwife who has been allocated to her. The notes should be checked for any specific instructions that have been laid down in the antenatal clinic. *High risk women* (see Appendix I) should be seen by the duty senior house officer (SHO) with the minimum of delay. After discussion with the duty registrar a plan of *Management for labour* should be made in the light of the antenatal instructions.

On admission the woman's temperature, pulse, blood pressure and the fetal heart rate should be recorded and the urine tested and the results entered on the partogram (see Section 1.3). An abdominal palpation should be performed and if the woman is thought to be in labour (and there are no contraindications) a vaginal examination should be performed and the results recorded as in Table 1.1.

A cardiotocographic recording (CTG) should be made on admission and should be of at least 20 min in length. The CTG must be inspected and signed soon after recording by a midwife or SHO trained to interpret CTGs, and filed securely in the patient's notes. The criteria for normality are found in Section 2.4.

If delivery is not imminent the woman should try to empty her bowels and should be offered a bath. It is not necessary to offer an enema routinely since this does not reduce the incidence of faecal soiling, but if she wishes the woman may have two glycerine suppositories. It is also unnecessary to shave the perineum since this has no effect upon the healing or infection rate of a vaginal or perineal wound.

1.3   MANAGEMENT OF LABOUR

Labour is diagnosed by the presence of regular, painful contractions which lead to progressive cervical change (effacement and dilatation).

1.4   THE FIRST STAGE OF LABOUR

This is defined as the period between the onset of labour and full dilatation of the cervix. Labour is monitored by means of a *partogram* which is a graphic record of the events which occur and of progress of labour. Its use aids continuity of care and helps the early recognition of abnormalities of labour.

The partogram should be started when the woman is admitted to the labour ward in suspected labour. The observations which should be recorded on the partogram are listed in Table 1.2 and detailed below.

Table 1.1   How to record a vaginal examination

1. Write in the notes in red ink and record the following:
   a.   The date, time and indication.
   b.   The abdominal findings, especially the number of fifths still palpable.
   c.   Whether catheterized. If so record the amount, and the presence or absence of ketones, protein and glucose.
   d.   The appearance of the external genitalia if this is the first vaginal examination.
   e.   The cervical dilatation (cm).
   f.   The degree of cervical effacement.
   g.   The state of the membranes.
   h.   The colour of the amniotic fluid.
   i.   The presenting part and its position.
   j.   The degree of moulding.
   k.   The details of any procedure performed, such as attaching a scalp clip.
2. An example:

   22/12/1986   0200 hour   Cephalic 1/5 palpable

   Vaginal examination to confirm full dilatation
   Cervix 9 cm. Absent membranes, clear amniotic fluid.
   Vertex presentation, ROP, moulding + +
   Scalp electrode re-applied.
3. Record the following findings on the partogram
   a.   Head level.
   b.   Cervical dilatation.

Table 1.2   Observations recorded on the partogram

Observation		Frequency
1.	Fetal heart rate	every 15 min
2.	Colour of amniotic fluid	hourly
3.	The fetal head level (fifths)	hourly
4.	The cervical dilatation	every 3–4 h
5.	The contractions (strength and frequency)	half-hourly
6.	Drugs (dose and route)	when given
7.	Syntocinon dosage (in dpm)	half-hourly
8.	Epidural top ups	when given
9.	Urine output	when passed
10.	Urine contents	with each specimen of urine
11.	Degree of moulding	at each vaginal examination
12.	Maternal BP and pulse	half-hourly
13.	Maternal temperature	half-hourly

1.4.1   Descent of the fetal head

Once labour is established an abdominal examination should be performed every 2 h to assess the descent of the fetal head, which is described as the number of fifths palpable above the pelvic brim (see Figure 1.1). The station of the fetal head in relation to the ischial spines is not recorded on the partogram because of the considerable inter-observer variation and because excessive caput succedaneum formation may give a false impression that the head is low.

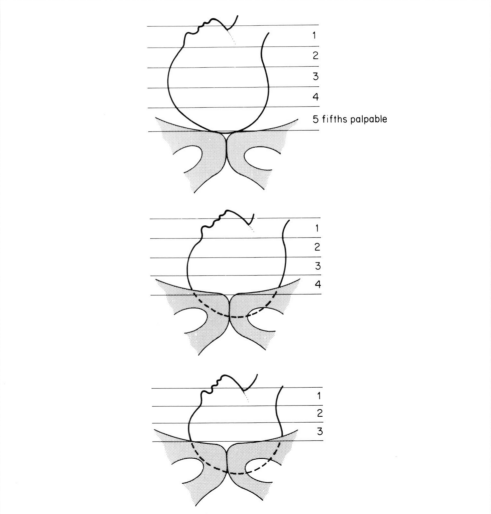

Figure 1.1   The method of determining head descent during labour. The amount of head that is palpable above the pelvic brim is in fifths. Abdominal palpation to determine the number of fifths still palpable should be made every 2 h and the result entered on the partogram. Failure of head descent is readily appreciable using this method

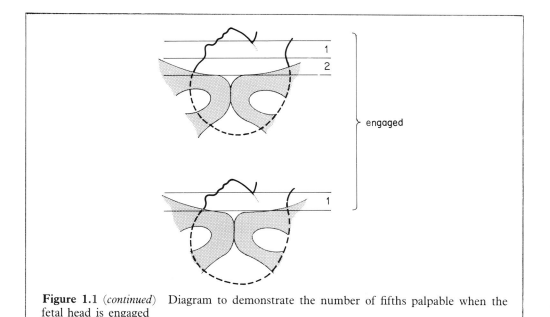

Figure 1.1 (*continued*)   Diagram to demonstrate the number of fifths palpable when the fetal head is engaged

1.4.2   Moulding

With descent of the fetal head a variable degree of overlapping of the bones of the fetal skull will occur, which is referred to as moulding. The significance of this is that an excessive degree of moulding implies cephalo–pelvic disproportion.

Moulding can be graded as follows:

0	No moulding
+	Parietal bones are closer together but do not touch
+ +	Parietal bones touch but do not overlap
+ + +	Parietal bones overlap but can be reduced
+ + + +	Irreducible overlapping of the parietal bones.

1.4.3   Cervical dilatation

Vaginal examinations are usually performed every 3–4 h to assess cervical dilatation. This examination may be performed by the midwife responsible for the care of the woman, or by the medical student or student midwife under appropriate supervision. Cervical dilatation is preceded by effacement or 'taking up' of the cervix. This is the process of shortening of the cervical canal and thinning of the cervix. In a multigravid patient, dilatation and effacement can occur simultaneously. The finding should be recorded as in Table 1.1.

Progress in labour demonstrated by cervical dilatation and descent of the fetal head is graphically recorded upon the partogram. Lines of expected or ideal progress have been derived by various workers (see Figure 1.2) and can be drawn on the partogram.

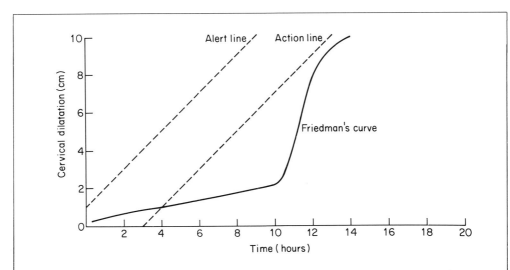

Figure 1.2   Lines of expected rates of progress of cervical dilatation. The solid curve is the first such curve derived but suffers from the disadvantage of starting from 0 cm of cervical dilatation. The dotted lines represent the alert and action lines devised by Philpott for African primigravidae. Patients were moved to hospital if they reached the alert line and stimulated with syntocinon if they reached the action line

A nomogram of cervical dilatation on admission to full dilatation to represent normal progress for patients in spontaneous labour is commercially available in the form of a stencil (Figure 1.3). The line of predicted progress can be drawn on the partogram according to the cervical dilatation on admission.

If cervical dilatation falls more than 2 h to the right of the nomogram it is considered to be abnormal and after vaginal examination to exclude a malpresentation a syntocinon infusion may be commenced (see Section 7.3.3).

1.4.4   Uterine contractions

These may be assessed in the following ways:

1. By progress in labour demonstrated by cervical effacement and dilatation. This is the only objective evidence of the efficiency of uterine activity.
2. By palpation—this provides a subjective impression of the strength of contractions together with the frequency and duration. Normal uterine contractions in the first stage of labour occur every 3–4 min, and last for 50–60 s.
    The way in which contractions should be recorded on the partogram is illustrated in Figure 1.4. Weak contractions are felt as very slight hardening of the uterus; moderate contractions when the uterine wall can still be indented by pressure with the thumb, and strong contractions when this is not possible.
3. By external tocography. This records the frequency and duration of uterine contractions. The recording of the baseline tone is inaccurate and the main purpose

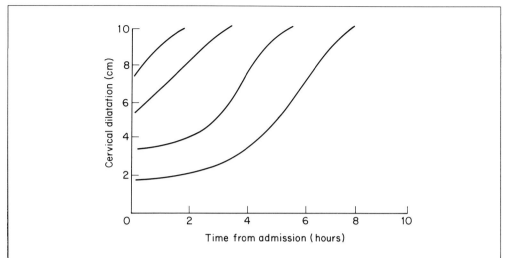

Figure 1.3   Nomograms of cervical dilatation rates (after Studd) representing expected progress in normal labour. More than 80 per cent of patients will progress on or to the right of the line drawn from the cervical dilatation on admission (Rocket and Co., Watford)

of such recordings is to relate changes in the fetal heart rate pattern to the contractions (see Chapter 2).

4. By means of an intra-uterine pressure catheter (IUC). This provides the most objective information about uterine activity. It will record the baseline tone, the frequency, duration and strength of uterine contractions together with information on uterine work. It is, however, an invasive procedure and is therefore only recommended in certain specific situations (see Section 8.4).

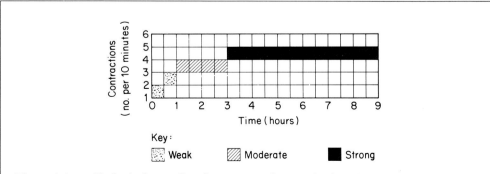

Figure 1.4   Method of recording frequency and strength of uterine contractions on the partogram

1.5 RUPTURE OF THE MEMBRANES

This is usually done in order to encourage progress in labour, to examine the colour of the amniotic fluid, and/or to attach a fetal scalp electrode. It should only be done when the fetal head is fully engaged and with a cervical dilatation of 4 cm or more. The membranes may be left intact when the woman does not wish them to be ruptured, providing that external fetal heart rate monitoring is technically adequate and the CTG trace is normal. Artificial rupture of the membranes (ARM) should be specifically recommended in the following instances:

1. Before the administration of syntocinon. The major hazard of the use of syntocinon with intact membranes is the risk of amniotic fluid embolism (see Section 16.5) and ARM should precede the syntocinon infusion. The exception to this rule is in the management of an intra-uterine death, when it is not advisable to perform ARM until labour is fully established because of the risk of intra-uterine infection (see Section 35.4).

    Rupturing the membranes will often encourage progress in labour, and therefore obviate the need for syntocinon.
2. To allow the application of a fetal scalp electrode which is indicated as follows:
    a. For any abnormality of the external CTG trace.
    b. If external monitoring is technically unsatisfactory.
    c. After rupture of membranes.
    d. If there is meconium staining of the amniotic fluid.
    e. In all high risk women (see Appendix I).

    If the woman wishes to be ambulant and there is a need for continuous monitoring, the telemetric CTG recording facility may be used.

1.6 AMBULATION AND POSITION IN LABOUR

In the first stage of labour many women wish to be ambulant. This may stimulate uterine activity, and although it does not reduce the length of labour, it increases the likelihood of spontaneous vaginal delivery. Many women are also more comfortable walking about in early labour.

Most women prefer to return to bed at approximately 6–7 cm of cervical dilatation. They should then be encouraged to lie on their side or should be well propped up in order to avoid the risks of supine hypotension. This is caused by the pressure of the uterus on the inferior vena cava and aorta, leading to reduced venous return and a fall in cardiac output and blood pressure. This is of particular importance for women with epidural anaesthesia (see Section 3.4).

1.7 FLUID BALANCE AND NUTRITION

Eating and drinking are not permitted during established labour because of the risks of vomiting and inhalation, particularly if general anaesthesia should be required. These risks result from delayed gastric emptying which is a feature of normal labour. Women are allowed sips of water or may suck on ice cubes. No other oral intake should be allowed once it has been decided that the woman is in labour.

All urine passed during labour should have its volume recorded and should be tested for glucose, protein and ketones. Micturition should be encouraged regularly particularly in women with epidural analgesia whose bladder sensation is impaired. These women should be offered a bed pan prior to each epidural top-up.

Ketonuria alone does not require correction in normal labour. If there is clinical evidence of dehydration, if there is fetal distress or if the uterine contractions are dysfunctional (see Section 8.2) then the woman should receive an intravenous infusion of Hartmann's solution or normal saline. Ketonuria does not represent starvation and the administration of dextrose, particularly 10 per cent, should not occur. The reason for this is that large volumes of electrolyte-free dextrose given intravenously can cause both maternal and neonatal hyponatraemia, with associated risks of neonatal apnoea, convulsions, respiratory distress and feeding difficulties. Maternal water intoxication is a further hazard if volumes of dextrose in excess of 3.5 l are given intravenously, particularly in association with oxytocic drugs and/or opiates both of which have anti-diuretic effects. In addition, in labour complicated by fetal acidosis administration of dextrose to the mother will provide further substrate to the fetus for anaerobic glycolysis thereby exacerbating lactic acidosis.

Therefore if the total i.v. fluid intake in any labour exceeds 3 l the registrar should be informed. Further fluid intake should be restricted, and if syntocinon is required its concentration can be doubled and the infusion rate halved.

1.8 THE SECOND STAGE OF LABOUR

1.8.1 Diagnosis

The second stage of labour is defined as the period between full dilatation of the cervix (10 cm) and delivery of the baby.

The diagnosis is made by vaginal examination. It may be suspected that the second stage has been reached when the woman experiences a reflex urge to push. The maternal anus will gape and the fetal head may become visible.

In certain situations the urge to push is felt before full dilatation of the cervix (e.g. in occipito–posterior position). It is almost impossible for the woman to voluntarily suppress this urge, and therefore appropriate analgesia must be given. If pushing continues, the cervix may become oedematous, a cervical tear may result and fetal distress often occurs. Epidural or other regional block is a very effective form of analgesia for this problem.

1.8.2 Management

When the woman has a strong desire to push and the second stage has been confirmed by vaginal examination she should be encouraged in her expulsive efforts. She should find a comfortable position but should not lie flat, thus avoiding the supine hypotension syndrome. The person conducting the delivery should be the only person giving instructions during pushing. Instructions from several different people will only serve to confuse the woman and increase her anxiety. Patients can only be taught to push effectively when they are in the second stage of labour.

Observations to be made throughout the second stage are listed on Table 1.3.

If uterine contractions are particularly weak or infrequent during the second stage, augmentation with syntocinon may be considered in primigravidae. This situation is unusual in multigravidae who should be reassessed to exclude obstructed labour (see Section 8.2).

Table 1.3 Observations made in the second stage of labour

	Observation	Frequency
1.	Maternal pulse and BP	every 30 min
2.	Contractions (strength and frequency)	continuously by palpation
3.	Fetal heart rate	continuously or after each contraction
4.	Maternal condition	continuously
5.	Maternal bladder size (by abdominal palpation)	at start of second stage

1.8.3 The length of the second stage

1.8.3.1 WITHOUT AN EPIDURAL

After full dilatation of the cervix and as soon as the woman experiences the urge to push she should be encouraged to do so. Effective pushing is usually allowed to continue for up to an hour in a primipara and half an hour in a multipara, after which time the duty registrar should assess the patient with a view to operative delivery. Other indications for considering operative delivery are maternal exhaustion or fetal distress (see Section 26.2).

1.8.3.2 WITH AN EPIDURAL

In these cases the second stage is more likely to be diagnosed by vaginal examination before the woman has the desire to push. Indeed no such desire may be experienced. Spontaneous delivery is more likely to occur if the fetal head is allowed to descend (and rotate) such that it is visible at the introitus before active pushing is commenced. In order for this to occur a further epidural top-up may be given in the second stage after which it is reasonable to wait a further 1–2 h, provided the maternal and fetal conditions are satisfactory.

It is cruel to allow the epidural to wear off fully in the second stage in a woman who has experienced a pain-free labour. To be exposed suddenly to second stage contractions is likely to cause extreme distress and the patient will be unable to maintain her composure or co-operate with instructions.

Given appropriate instructions a woman is able to push effectively whilst she has full analgesia from an epidural block.

Effective pushing may continue for up to an hour in a primiparous woman or 30 min in multiparous woman. After this time, instrumental delivery should be considered (see Section 26.2).

1.9   THE THIRD STAGE OF LABOUR

This is defined as the period between delivery of the baby and delivery of the placenta.

1.9.1   Management

1. One ampoule of syntometrine (5 units of syntocinon and 500 µg of ergometrine) should be given by intramuscular injection to the mother with the delivery of the anterior shoulder of the fetus (or with the crowning of the head in breech presentation) except in the following circumstances:
    a. Hypertension: a blood pressure equal to or greater than 140/90 mmHg. This is because ergometrine has α-adrenergic properties and so causes peripheral vasoconstriction, increased venous return and elevation of blood pressure. Syntometrine is replaced by 5 units of syntocinon i.v.
    b. Maternal cardiac disease (see Chapter 28).
    c. The first of twins (see Chapter 18). Syntometrine is given as above with the delivery of the second twin.
    d. When the woman refuses it. In this case the refusal should be documented in the case notes after the full risks of postpartum haemorrhage and its consequences have been explained. Ideally the subject should have been discussed antenatally.
2. The cord should be clamped within 15 s (or as soon as possible) after delivery to avoid an excessive transfusion of blood from the placenta to the neonate, which may result in a hyperviscosity syndrome with associated problems. After the cord is clamped and divided the placenta should be delivered by controlled cord traction. If clamping is refused, the baby should be kept at the same level as the placenta, to avoid an excessive placento-fetal transfusion.
3. Umbilical cord blood should be taken if necessary (see Appendix III).
4. All women whose labours have been augmented with syntocinon should continue to receive the infusion for at least 1 h after delivery. If the woman is at high risk of postpartum haemorrhage a prophylactic regimen of syntocinon should be instituted (see Section 13.3).
5. If an episiotomy was performed or a tear was sustained, repair should take place as soon as possible (see Section 4.4).

1.10   WHEN LABOUR IS NOT DIAGNOSED

A woman may suspect she is in labour, but after a period of time this is found not to be the case. Observations, including monitoring of the fetal heart for at least 20 min should be performed. If these are satisfactory, and no cervical changes are observed over a reasonable period of time (at least 2 h), the situation should be reassessed. Some women experience a very painful latent stage of labour. This refers to the period up to 3 cm of cervical dilatation, and when it lasts several hours strong analgesia may be required (see Section 8.2).

If the woman complains of a symptom such as abdominal pain, which is not immediately explicable, or suggests the possibility of complications, admission, observation and investigation may be appropriate. If she has no unexplained symptoms and observations are satisfactory, then she may be allowed home with appropriate follow-up arrangements made.

Chapter 2

Intrapartum Fetal Heart Monitoring

2.1 INTRODUCTION

Controversy continues to surround the universal application of fetal heart rate monitoring in labour. Opponents argue that it is an unnecessary encumbrance to the mother, resulting in an unduly high rate of intervention. On the other hand, if abnormalities of the fetal heart rate (FHR) are recognized promptly and dealt with appropriately, fetal asphyxia and therefore perinatal morbidity and mortality can be reduced.

2.1.1 Limitations of auscultation with the Pinard stethoscope

1. Abnormalities of baseline variability (see below) and/or shallow decelerations cannot be perceived by the human ear.
2. There is a tendency for the observer to calculate the fetal heart rate by rounding up or down to the nearest five or ten. The shorter the period of auscultation, the greater the inaccuracy of the result.
3. Counting the FHR results is an *average* rate, rather than an *instantaneous* rate.
4. Auscultation is only intermittent, and therefore abnormalities may occur when no monitoring is taking place.
5. Auscultation may be technically difficult if the woman prefers an alternative position in labour.

6.   Unless auscultation takes place immediately after a contraction, significant fetal heart decelerations may be missed.

Staff should be trained to use a Pinard stethoscope whilst monitoring the fetal heart rate electronically. This leads to more accurate use of the Pinard stethoscope, and to the practice of periodically checking the monitor by means of the Pinard's stethoscope is to be be encouraged.

2.2   MONITORING POLICIES

Hospital policy on intrapartum fetal heart monitoring will depend to a certain extent upon the financial constraints which limit the availability of CTG monitors. If there are enough monitors every woman may be offered intrapartum fetal heart monitoring. Alternative policies include:

1.   Monitoring only high risk women (see Appendix I).
2.   Monitoring all high risk women and some low risk women.

The CTG tracing, however, should be regarded as a screening test. Normal patterns are reassuring but even the most suspicious fetal heart rate patterns may not be associated with fetal asphyxia, and CTG monitoring should be supported by fetal scalp pH determination (see Section 15.5).

2.3   TECHNIQUE OF FETAL HEART RATE MONITORING (FHRM)

2.3.1   External FHRM

The transducer used to detect the FHR utilizes the Doppler principle, whereby emitted ultrasound waves undergo a shift in frequency after reflection by a moving structure such as the fetal heart. The FHR is thus monitored by detection of mechanical rather than electrical energy.

1.   Advantages of external monitoring:
     a.   It can be used whilst membranes are still intact.
     b.   It does not involve attaching a clip to the fetal head.
2.   Disadvantages:
     a.   Most machines average every three heart beats therefore beat-to-beat variation cannot be assessed.
     b.   The quality of the tracing depends upon the patient being relatively immobile. Movement will lead to artifact.
     c.   Technical problems may lead to ultrasonic doubling or halving of the fetal heart rate.
     d.   It is not possible to use this technique for simultaneous FHRM of twins (see Section 18.3) as the two Doppler transducers interfere with each other's signal.

The external CTG may be recorded in early labour and if the tracing is considered normal it may be discontinued for 4 h, or until the woman needs analgesia or returns to bed, whichever occurs first.

If the external CTG is considered abnormal (see Section 15.4) then ARM and application of a fetal scalp electrode (FSE) is necessary.

2.3.2 Internal FHRM

The fetal scalp electrode (FSE) detects the electrical energy produced during each cardiac cycle. Fetal heart monitors are usually designed to be triggered by the R wave of the fetal ECG. The monitor is able to process the incoming signals and compare them to earlier signals, providing a precise instantaneous recording of the FHR so allowing assessment of baseline variability.

If the woman expresses any reluctance to ARM and application of a FSE, external monitoring may continue provided the tracing is satisfactory. However, internal monitoring should be specifically recommended in the following instances:

1. All high risk women (see Appendix I).
2. Any abnormality of the external CTG trace.
3. Meconium-staining of the amniotic fluid.
4. Women with epidural analgesia.
5. Breech presentation (in this situation care should be taken to apply the electrode to a buttock or foot).

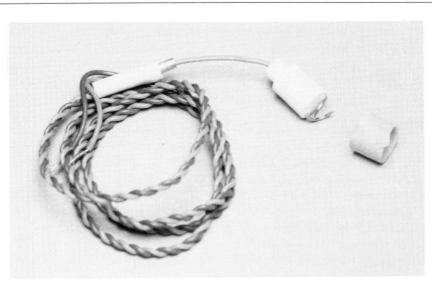

Figure 2.1   A spiral electrode. These are applied by means of an applicator

6.   All patients receiving syntocinon augmentation.
7.   Multiple pregnancy (see Section 18.3).

   Ideally a Copeland electrode (Figure 2.2) is used rather than a single spiral electrode (Figure 2.1), and care is taken during application to place it over the parietal bone of the fetal scalp, avoiding the anterior and posterior fontanelles.
   If the woman wishes to remain mobile she may do so if telemetry (Figure 2.3) is available.

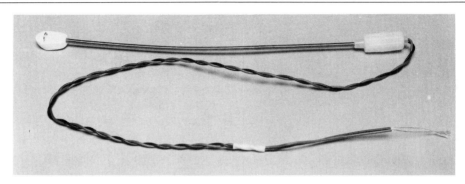

Figure 2.2   A Copeland electrode. The electrode is applied to the fetal head by rotating the far end which withdraws the semi-circular wire. Once the electrode is pushed tightly against the fetal head the far end is released to allow the semi-circular wire to penetrate the infant's scalp

2.4 NORMAL CTG

A normal CTG (Figure 2.4) has the following characteristics:

1.   A fetal heart rate of 120–160 beats min^{-1}.
2.   No decelerations of the fetal heart rate.
3.   Baseline variability of 5–15 beats min^{-1}.

   Accelerations of the FHR with contractions are a sign of a healthy fetus (see Figure 2.4), but their absence in advanced labour is not a poor prognostic sign.

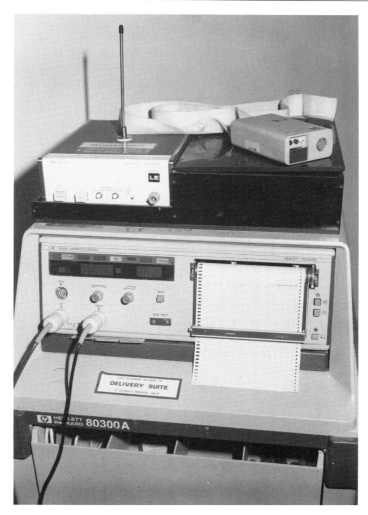

Figure 2.3 A fetal heart rate monitor that allows the use of telemetry. The small apparatus on top of the black box is carried in a sling by the women and receives the signal directly from the tocograph and from the scalp electrode. This is transmitted to the aerial on the left hand side of the monitor. Effective range is 20–30 m

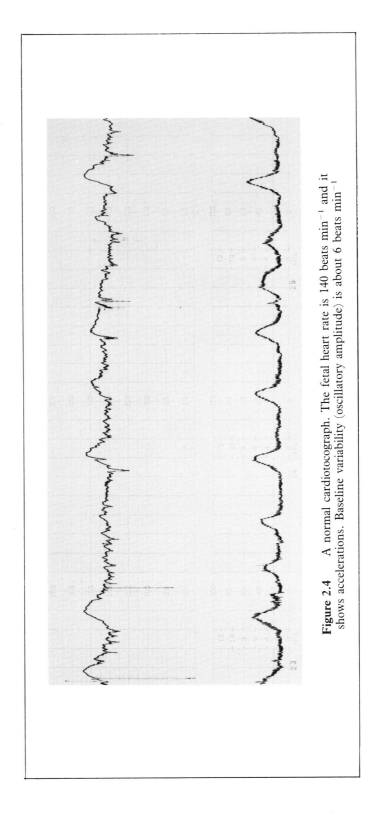

Figure 2.4   A normal cardiotocograph. The fetal heart rate is 140 beats min^{-1} and it shows accelerations. Baseline variability (oscillatory amplitude) is about 6 beats min^{-1}

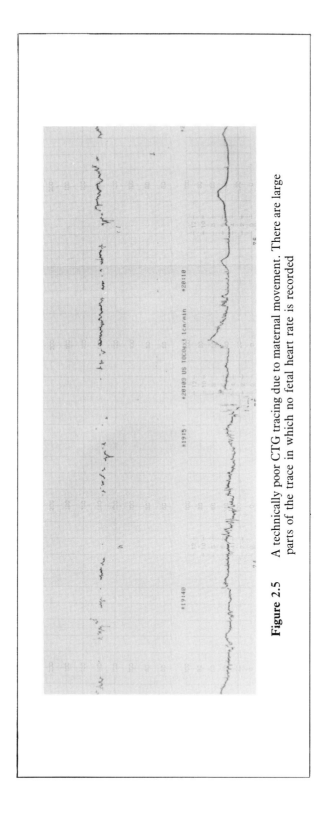

Figure 2.5   A technically poor CTG tracing due to maternal movement. There are large parts of the trace in which no fetal heart rate is recorded

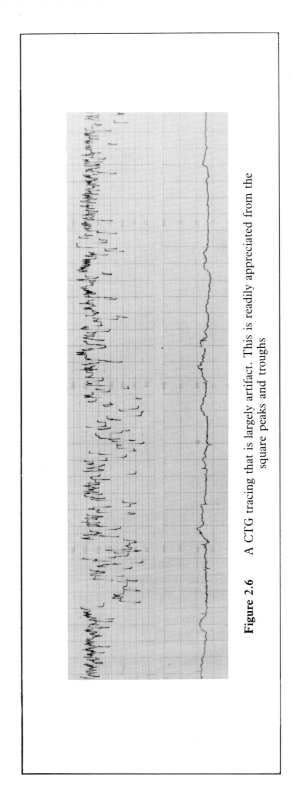

Figure 2.6   A CTG tracing that is largely artifact. This is readily appreciated from the square peaks and troughs

2.5   COMMON ERRORS IN FETAL HEART MONITORING

1. Poor signals, leading to a technically poor tracing which cannot be interpreted (Figure 2.5).
2. Failure to record contractions, leading to inability to interpret significance of decelerations.
3. Artefact (Figure 2.6).
4. Failure to recognize when the signal recorded is the maternal heart rate. This phenomenon can occur with either external or internal monitoring.
5. Failure to recognize a sinusoidal pattern and the more subtle abnormalities of baseline variability (see Section 15.4).
6. Failure to write on the trace and record significant events namely:
   a. *Name, date and time.*
   b. Position or change of position of the patient.
   c. Drugs given.
   d. Administration of an epidural and subsequent top-ups.
   e. Vaginal examinations.
   f. Onset of second stage of labour.
   g. Onset of pushing.

Chapter 3
Analgesia and Anaesthesia

3.1 INTRODUCTION

The alleviation of severe pain during labour is desirable for several reasons. Firstly it allows childbirth to be enjoyed by the woman and her partner. Secondly severe pain results in fear and anxiety which increases maternal catecholamine release resulting in inefficient uterine action and prolonged labour. Thus a vicious circle known as the pain–fear–anxiety syndrome is set up (see Section 8.1).

A painful and prolonged labour is an almost universal fear by pregnant women as they approach term. Much of the anxiety surrounding the prospect of labour can be allayed by antenatal education and instruction. This should include discussion of available forms of analgesia. The beneficial effect of a constant companion in labour is well-proven, and the support and trust which develops between the woman and a good midwife may lessen the need for strong analgesia. Unforseen events occurring during labour may result in a medical indication for a particular form of analgesia for the benefit of mother and/or fetus, but the choice, as ever, is ultimately with the patient. A sense of guilt is unfortunately not unusual, when a woman has been led to believe that analgesia is unnecessary and subsequently requires pain relief.

3.2   NARCOTIC ANALGESICS

Pethidine may be given in the first stage of labour as an intramuscular injection in doses from 50 mg to 150 mg at intervals of 3–4 h. Around 40–60 per cent of patients will experience some pain relief after 100 mg. Most women experience slight euphoria, with nausea, vomiting, dizziness and agitation the most frequent side-effects, so it is usually administered with an antiemetic such as stemetil 12.5 mg i.m. Rarely, maternal hypotension and respiratory depression occur. All narcotics further delay gastric emptying and reduce the tone of the gasto-oesophageal sphincter, hence increasing the risk of inhalation if general anaesthesia becomes necessary.

Pethidine is readily transferred to the fetus, and respiratory depression can be expected if delivery occurs between 1 h and 3 h of its administration. Neonatal effects are rarely seen if delivery occurs within 20 min of maternal administration. The half-life of the drug in the neonate is six times that in the adult. To avoid the risk of neonatal respiratory depression, it is unusual to give more than two doses of pethidine during labour. If the need for further analgesia arises, an epidural block should be considered.

Morphine, omnopon and *diamorphine* are more potent analgesics, but have more profound respiratory depressant effects on the neonate. Their use is therefore usually restricted to labours following fetal death.

The respiratory depressant effects of all narcotic agents on the fetus may be effectively reversed by *naloxone hydrochloride* (Narcan) at a dose of 0.5–1.0 ml for preterm infants and 1.0–2.0 ml for term infants, by intramuscular injection.

Meptazinol (Meptid) 100 mg by intramuscular injection has been promoted as a more effective alternative to pethidine, with less nausea and vomiting, but this remains to be substantiated.

3.2   INHALATION ANALGESIA

Inhalation analgesia is used intermittently in the latter part of the first stage (transitional phase) and early second stage, and may provide rapid and efficient pain relief. A non-rebreathing apparatus fitted either with a mask or mouth-piece (Figure 3.1) delivers a fixed concentration of the agent, which is self-administered, beginning when the contraction is first palpated by the attendant midwife. Contractions are usually felt by an observer some 15–30 s before the women becomes aware of them and this is sufficient time for the agent to be inhaled and to act on the maternal brain.

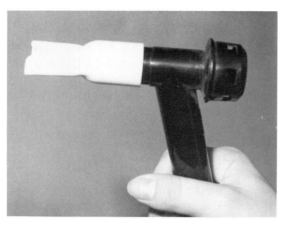

Figure 3.1   A mouth piece suitable for the self administration of inhalation analgesia. Many patients find this preferable to an anaesthetic face mask which commonly has a rubbery smell and may induce feelings of suffocation

Nitrous oxide is most commonly used in a 50 per cent concentration in oxygen (Entonox) and is free from any maternal cardio-respiratory depressive effect and has no fetal effects. Disadvantages of this form of pain relief are that hyperventilation is occasionally encouraged if the woman is not properly instructed, and tearfulness and/ or excitation are sometimes seen with over-usage. The technique of breathing Entonox prevents the use of breathing techniques used in 'natural childbirth'.

Trichloroethylene is little used because of its cumulative sedative effect upon both mother and fetus, effects which are shared by *methoxyflurane*.

3.4 EPIDURAL ANAESTHESIA

This form of analgesia is achieved by the injection of a local anaesthetic agent into the epidural space. This space is entered through a lumbar intervertebral space (Figure 3.2). Complete anaesthesia for labour and vaginal delivery requires a block from T10 to S5 (Figure 3.3). For a Caesarean section under epidural, a block from T6 to S1 is necessary.

This form of pain relief should ideally be available on request at any time of the day or night, by an experienced anaesthetist of at least registrar grade.

The advantages of epidural anaesthesia are that it provides excellent analgesia in most women with a very low incidence of maternal and fetal complications. If operative delivery is necessary later, (either vaginal or abdominal) the woman has the option of delivery under epidural. In the first stage of labour an epidural may encourage progress by abolishing pain and anxiety and allowing both physical and psychological recovery.

The disadvantages include variable loss of motor function of the lower limbs, and bladder dysfunction.

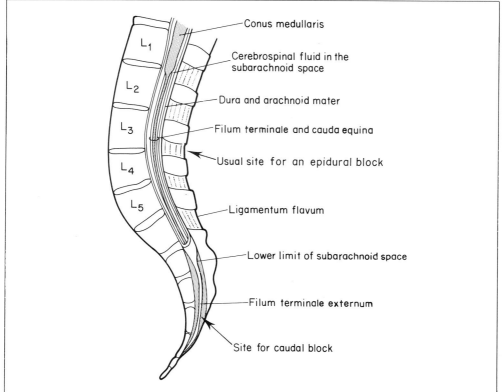

Figure 3.2   The anatomy of the epidural space in the lumbosacral region. The epidural cannula is usually sited at the L3/4 level. Caudal analgesia is administered through the sacral hiatus whilst a spinal anaesthetic involves piercing the dura mater such that the anaesthetic agent is put into the cerebrospinal fluid

The incidence of forceps delivery after an epidural block is increased, particularly in primigravidae. This is due to relaxation of pelvic floor muscles which normally assist in rotation of the fetal head, decreased oxytocin release and by reduction of the bearing-down reflex and the efficiency of maternal expulsive efforts. The likelihood of a forceps delivery can be minimized if a policy of delayed pushing is adopted (see Section 1.8). The duration of pushing in women who achieve spontaneous delivery is not prolonged by this policy, neither is there an increase in fetal distress.

The effects of extradural injection of local anaesthetic drugs produces both parasympathetic and sympathetic blockade, resulting in difficulty in micturition and hypotension respectively. *Bupivicaine* (Marcain) is the preferred drug because it has a longer duration than lignocaine and is three to four times more potent with less placental transfer. Various concentrations from 0.125 per cent to 0.5 per cent solution are used as intermittent injections, producing analgesia for 1–3 h. Recently, continuous low dose infusions by syringe pump have become popular.

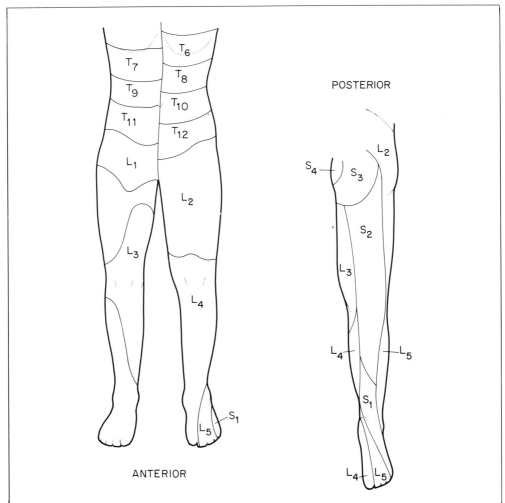

Figure 3.3   Dermatomes. In order to achieve a pain free labour and delivery it is necessary to block the nerves supplying T10 to S5. If Caesarean section is to be performed using epidural anaesthesia the block must extend to T6 to prevent the patient being aware of the surgeon pulling on the peritoneum

3.4.1   Absolute contraindications

1.   Patient refusal.
2.   Local sepsis.
3.   Anticoagulant therapy or a bleeding diathesis, because of the possibility of extradural haemorrhage resulting in paraplegia.
4.   Inadequate staffing. All women with epidural analgesia must have a midwife present continually.
5.   Certain cardiac diseases e.g. obstructive cardiomyopathy, where the reduction in

venous return secondary to peripheral vasodilation may be fatal (see also Chapter 28).

3.4.2 Relative contraindications

1. Severe supine hypotension. If an epidural is needed in such patients a pre-load of 500 ml of Hartmann's solution and avoidance of the supine position usually overcome the problem.
2. Severe or fulminating pre-eclampsia. This may pose the following problems:
   a. Profound hypotension. Patients with pre-eclampsia have a reduced plasma volume and sympathetic blockade caused by the epidural together with antihypertensive agents may cause a marked fall in blood pressure. A pre-load of 500 ml Hartmann's solution, and a reduced dose of antihypertensive, are therefore necessary.
   b. If the patient has a disseminated intravascular coagulopathy (DIC) an epidural haematoma may result. Normal clotting function (see Section 14.3) should be confirmed before administering the epidural.
3. Neurological disease, e.g. multiple sclerosis. In this instance subsequent neurological deterioration may be attributed by the patient to the administration of an epidural. If the patient understands, after a full explanation by the anaesthetist, that there is little risk that an epidural will increase the rate of deterioration of her disease then she may be allowed to have one. A note to the effect that this agreement has taken place should be recorded in the case notes.
4. A history of back injury or laminectomy. This needs careful discussion with the consultant anaesthetist before an epidural is considered.

3.4.3 Indications

Epidural anaesthesia is positively indicated in the following situations:

1. Maternal request.
2. Dysfunctional labour, particularly where narcotic analgesia has been unhelpful, and/or in those patients with occipito–posterior position of the fetal head.
3. Breech presentation (see Chapter 19).
4. Multiple pregnancy (see Chapter 18).
5. Preterm labour (see Chapter 9).
6. Maternal diabetes mellitus (see Chapter 27).
7. Maternal cardiac disease (except aortic stenosis and hypertrophic obstructive cardiomyopathy—see Chapter 28).

3.4.4 Management

The following procedure should be adopted:

1. When the epidural is indicated for obstetric reasons the duty obstetric registrar should discuss the case with the anaesthetist. This is particularly important in cases of pre-eclampsia, stillbirth or fetal anomaly.
2. All women must have an intravenous infusion running via a 14 gauge cannula before the epidural is set up and should receive a pre-load of 500 ml of Hartmann's solution over 20 min before the epidural is commenced.
3. If the anaesthetic registrar twice fails to insert the epidural or takes longer than 10 min then he should call the senior registrar or duty consultant.
4. *Topping-up* the epidural may be performed by a midwife or SHO who has received appropriate instruction in the procedure (see below). The anaesthetist's directions as to dose and position during and immediately after top-up should be followed. The midwife must never give the first test dose of Marcain.

It is not the place of this book to describe the techniques of insertion of an epidural cannula. The reader is referred to textbooks of anaesthesia.

3.4.5   Procedure for epidural top-up

1. As soon as the patient begins to feel discomfort with contractions the epidural should be topped-up. Top-ups should not be delayed as it is easier to prevent pain than treat it.
2. Ampoules with the correct concentrations of Marcain of ampoules should be selected.
3. The midwife or SHO should wash their hands and draw up the required dose, again checking the ampoule and written instructions with a second person.
4. After attaching the syringe with Marcain to the end of the epidural cannula, it should be aspirated through the two-way bacterial filter before injecting the Marcain. If more than 0.5 ml of fluid can be aspirated the anaesthetist is informed immediately, and the Marcain is withheld since this may suggest a dural tap.
5. The Marcain should be injected slowly through the filter, and the cap covering it is replaced at the end of the procedure. Injection should not occur during a contraction.
6. The woman's blood pressure and pulse rate and the fetal heart rate are recorded immediately after the top-up, and then recorded every 5 min for half an hour.
7. Hypotension may occur as a result of sympathetic blockade and vasodilation of the lower limbs. It may be accompanied by FHR decelerations of varying amplitudes. In this event, the woman should be placed on her left side and 1 ℓ of Hartmann's solution should be given intravenously over 15–20 min whilst medical assistance is summoned. If the FHR abnormality persists oxygen should be administered by face mask at 4 ℓ min^{-1} and a fetal blood sample considered. If the hypotension does not resolve within 10 min the anaesthetist should be recalled, and 1 ℓ of Haemaccel should be infused.
8. Patients should generally be offered a bed pan prior to each top-up. This is the time when they have most bladder sensation and are more likely to void spontaneously.
9. *The midwife must inform the anaesthetist immediately if she is concerned about the*

woman's condition or if the epidural is not working correctly. Inadequate analgesia may often be overcome by top-ups in appropriate positions but if this fails the epidural should be re-sited.

10. After delivery, the midwife responsible for the woman should remove the epidural catheter and carefully examine it. The time of removal of the catheter and the fact that it is complete should be recorded in the notes.

3.4.6   Complications of epidural anaesthesia

3.4.6.1   BLADDER DYSFUNCTION

If the woman is offered a bed pan prior to a top-up she may void urine spontaneously. Prior to each vaginal examination the abdomen should be palpated to detect bladder distension. If the woman is unable to void spontaneously a disposable plastic catheter should be inserted and the bladder drained and the catheter removed. If a second catheterization is required, however, this should be with a 10 or 12 French gauge Foley catheter with a 5–10 ml balloon. The catheter should normally be removed at the end of labour but if this occurs late at night it may be removed at 6 a.m. the next morning.

Any woman who has not voided urine within 6 h of a labour associated with an epidural or 6 h after removal of the Foley catheter should be reported to the duty SHO immediately. Recatheterization will be necessary if the patient is in acute retention either by the urethral or suprapubic route. If the retention is painless the patient should have a full neurological assessment.

3.4.6.2   DURAL TAP

Procedure to be followed in the event of a dural puncture occurring during the administration of an epidural block for pain relief in labour.

1. The anaesthetist should withdraw Tuohy needle and call a more senior anaesthetist to continue the procedure if possible.
2. The senior anaesthetist should be called upon to ensure the woman has an effective epidural, since she will require an elective forceps delivery to avoid the need for pushing in second stage of labour. The epidural will be sited one space higher.
3. The anaesthetist should write an account in the patient's notes and inform the obstetric team. The consultant obstetric anaesthetist should also be informed.
4. The patient should be nursed in the supine position for 24 h after delivery. If she has no headache after that time she may be mobilized.
5. If headache is present paracetamol (1 g) every 4–5 h may be given until the pain is relieved.
6. If headache persists beyond 48 h the patient should be kept supine until it has gone.
7. The patient should be kept well hydrated. Continue intravenous fluids for 24 h and ensure a total input of at least 3 ℓ day^{-1} of fluid.
8. Laxatives must be given routinely, as straining increases headache.

9. The person responsible for the dural tap must visit the patient every day until the headache has gone.
10. If the headache persists for more than 5 days consider an epidural 'blood patch' where a few millilitres of the patient's blood is injected into the epidural space, but only after discussion with consultant anaesthetist.

3.4.6.3 INCOMPLETE ANALGESIA

Occasionally the patient experiences inadequate over-all analgesia, or continued pain in one particular site or on one particular side. This can sometimes be overcome by alterations of position of the patient during top-ups, as advised by the anaesthetist.

3.5 CAUDAL ANAESTHESIA

This is a very low epidural where the cannula pierces the sacral hiatus (Figure 3.2), thus entering the lowest part of the epidural space. It is occasionally used as analgesia for instrumental delivery. It is usually given as a single shot by the anaesthetist or obstetrician concerned. The patient's blood pressure should be recorded at 5 min intervals for the next 15 min. Otherwise no special observations or care are required.

3.5.1 Complications

3.5.1.1 FAILURE

This occurs in about 5 per cent of cases and is usually due to the extremely variable anatomy of the sacro-coccygeal junction.

3.5.1.2 DURAL TAP

This should not occur if the needle used is less than 4 cm in length.

3.5.1.3 PENETRATION OF MATERNAL RECTUM AND/OR FETAL SCALP

Again this is avoided by using needles of less than 4 cm in length.

3.6 SPINAL ANAESTHESIA

This is achieved by the introduction of a local anaesthetic into the subarachnoid space (Figure 3.2). A level of block to the tenth thoracic dermatome (T10) will produce analgesia during labour. A slightly higher level of block to T6 is necessary for analgesia for Caesarean section.

Spinal anaesthesia is an alternative to pudendal block for forceps delivery if the patient has not had an epidural or caudal block. It may also be used for manual removal of the placenta.

3.6.1 Complications

3.6.1.1 HYPOTENSION

This can usually be reversed with a rapid infusion of 500 ml of Hartmann's solution.

3.6.1.2 TOTAL SPINAL BLOCKADE

Respiratory paralysis may occur if an excessive dose of local anaesthetic has been administered. The hypotension should be treated with intravenous fluids and if necessary endotracheal intubation and artificial ventilation should be started. Elevation of the legs will assist venous return. This risk is small in the hands of well-trained personnel.

3.6.1.3 SPINAL HEADACHE

This may last for up to six days and is worse on standing. It is caused by leakage of cerebrospinal fluid from the puncture site of the meninges. It occurs in only about 0.5 per cent of patients when small (26 gauge) needles are used.

3.6.1.4 BLADDER DYSFUNCTION

Observations are as for epidural anaesthesia.

3.7 LOCAL ANAESTHESIA

A pudendal block generally provides rather poor anaesthesia for midcavity forceps delivery but is frequently used when the woman has not already been given epidural, spinal or caudal anaesthesia and when delivery is urgent. Outlet forceps deliveries when the fetal head is on the perineum, can usually be satisfactorily accomplished by local infiltration of the perineum along the site of the episiotomy. A pudendal block does not provide sufficient analgesia for a rotational forceps delivery.

Plain lignocaine 1 per cent (10 mg ml^{-1}) is completely adequate for both pudendal block and perineal anaesthesia. The maximal dose should be 7 mg kg^{-1} or about 400 mg (40 ml of 1 per cent plain lignocaine).

3.7.1 Technique of pudendal block

The operator inserts the index and middle fingers of his left hand into the space between the fetal head and the lateral vaginal wall until he locates the ischial spine. A pudendal needle guard (see Figure 3.4) is then guided along between the operator's middle and index finger until it reaches the vagina covering the ischial spine (Figure 3.5). The needle is inserted down the guard and 10 ml of 1 per cent plain lignocaine are injected after aspiration. The procedure is repeated on the other side. As this technique does not block the skin innervated by the posterior cutaneous nerves of the thigh (see Figure 3.6) the line of the proposed episiotomy must also be infiltrated with 10 ml of 1 per cent plain lignocaine.

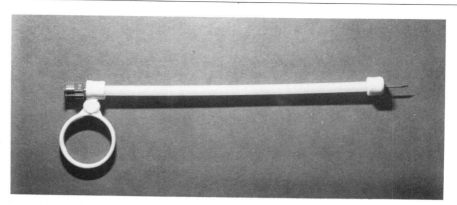

Figure 3.4   A pudendal needle with its guard. The guard prevents the needle from being inserted to a depth of more than 1 cm

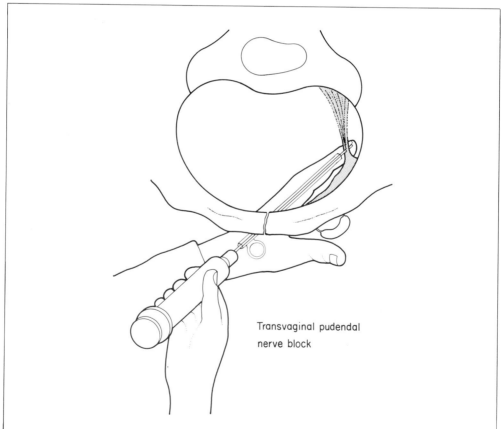

Transvaginal pudendal
nerve block

Figure 3.5   Diagram of method of performing a transvaginal pudendal nerve block

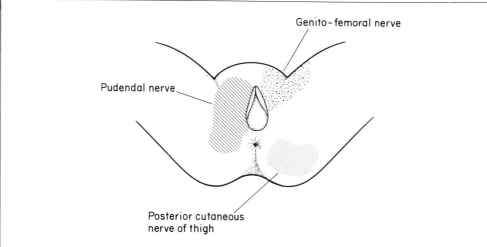

Figure 3.6   The innervation of the female perineum. Note that the pudendal nerve (S2, 3, 4) does not supply all the skin in the line of the episiotomy. The lower part is supplied by the posterior cutaneous nerve of thigh

3.8   GENERAL ANAESTHESIA

The major hazard of general anaesthesia in pregnancy is the risk of aspiration of the gastric contents resulting in a chemical pneumonitis (Mendelson's syndrome or pulmonary aspiration syndrome).

This is more likely to occur in pregnancy due to delay in gastric emptying, which is more evident during labour and after narcotic analgesia (but not after an epidural). During induction of anaesthesia passive regurgitation may occur due to relaxation of the gastro-oesophageal sphincter and raised intra-gastric pressure. The crico-pharyngeal sphincter is paralysed by skeletal muscle relaxants, so regurgitated gastric contents can easily reach the pharynx. The treatment is described in Section 16.7.

3.8.1.   Prevention of Mendelson's syndrome of pulmonary aspiration

1. The anaesthetist should be sufficiently experienced and competent to administer a general anaesthetic to an obstetric patient.
2. Eating or drinking large volumes of fluid are not permitted during labour.
3. Antacid prophylaxis should be given to reduce gastric acidity, and therefore minimize pulmonary reaction should aspiration occur. Recommended regimens are as follows:
    a. Elective Caesarean section
        (i)   Ranitidine 150 mg orally the night prior to surgery.
        (ii) Ranitidine 150 mg orally (with a small sip of water) 2 h pre-operatively.
        (iii) 30 ml 0.3 M sodium citrate immediately prior to the general anaesthetic.

    b. Emergency Caesarean section
       (i) Ranitidine 150 mg orally when blood is sent for cross-matching.
      (ii) 30 ml 0.3 M sodium citrate before being taken to theatre.
    c. Women at high risk of operative delivery. (e.g. Trial of scar, breech presentation, etc.) These should receive 150 mg Ranitidine every 6 h in labour and 0.3 M sodium citrate immediately pre-operatively.

4. Endotracheal intubation is mandatory.

5. Pressure should be applied to the cricoid cartilage by an assistant from the beginning of induction until the cuff of the tube is inflated.

6. There should be a recognized 'failed intubation drill' to follow.

3.8.2   Awareness during anaesthesia

In order to minimize the effect of intravenous induction agents and analgesic drugs upon the fetus, a very light plane of narcosis is the aim in obstetric anaesthesia in a totally paralysed patient. Occasionally maternal awareness of intra-operative events can occur, with later recall, or of the memory of an unpleasant dream. Maintenance of anaesthesia with a low concentration of an inhalation agent such as halothane may decrease the risk of this phenomenon as may the use of agents causing amnesia (e.g. diazepam) which can be administered to the mother after the delivery of the baby. If the patient complains of such awareness it should be explained to her that the light anaesthetic was necessary for the baby's sake.

Chapter 4
Episiotomy

4.1 DEFINITION

An episiotomy is a deliberate incision of the vagina and perineum to facilitate delivery of the fetal head.

4.2 INDICATIONS

1. Fetal distress—when the perineum is seen to be delaying delivery.
2. Preterm delivery (see Section 9.9).
3. Imminent tearing. The assessment of when this is likely should be left to the discretion of the person performing the delivery. One of the difficulties is that it is almost impossible to predict the extent and severity of a tear, but this does not mean that routine episiotomies are justified.
4. A rigid, scarred perineum.

5. An anterior episiotomy is likely to be necessary after female circumcision, often encountered with Sudanese women.
6. Instrumental delivery usually necessitates an episiotomy. Occasionally, when a Ventouse extraction is performed for delay in the second stage, an episiotomy may be unnecessary.
7. Previous third degree tear.
8. Breech delivery.
9. Twin delivery.

4.3   TYPES OF EPISIOTOMY

See Figure 4.1.

1. Midline.
2. J-shaped.
3. Mediolateral.

Advantages of midline episiotomies:

1. Healing is better.
2. Repair is easier and a good anatomical result is easier to achieve.
3. Bleeding is reduced.
4. It is less painful in the puerperium and leads to earlier resumption of intercourse.

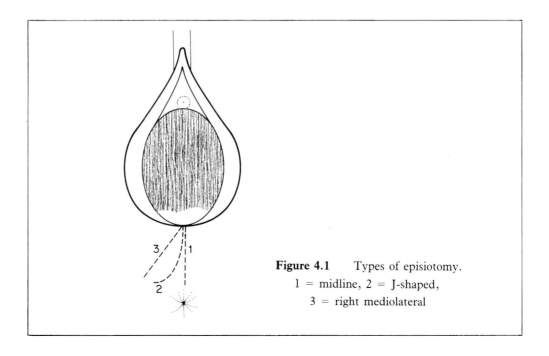

Figure 4.1   Types of episiotomy.
1 = midline, 2 = J-shaped,
3 = right mediolateral

The disadvantages of midline episiotomies are that they may (about twice as frequently as other episiotomies) extend to third degree tears, involving the anal sphincter, and occasionally the rectal mucosa.

In many hospitals the mediolateral episiotomy is therefore the preferred type.

4.3.1 Technique

In all but urgent cases the proposed episiotomy and the indication should be explained to the woman and her verbal consent obtained. Between contractions the skin and underlying muscle along the line of the proposed episiotomy should be infiltrated with at least 10 ml of 1 per cent plain lignocaine (see Figure 3.5) unless there is an effective epidural block. The episiotomy should be cut when the presenting part is distending the perineum.

The incision should be made with scissors commencing from the midline of the fourchette (see Figure 4.2). The fingers of the operator protect the presenting part of the baby.

4.4 PRINCIPLES OF REPAIR

1. The suturing should be performed as soon as possible after delivery, by someone appropriately trained or supervised.

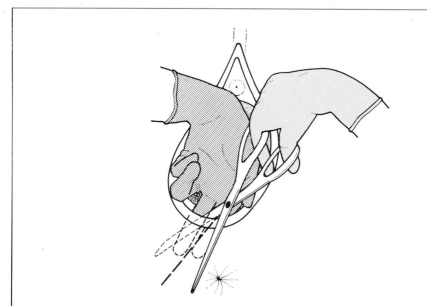

Figure 4.2 Technique of cutting an episiotomy. The middle and index finger of the operator's left hand are inserted into the vagina and protect the presenting part and the vagina from the scissors

2. Adequate analgesia is essential. If the woman has been given an epidural it should be topped-up before the repair.
3. Good visualization of the tear or episiotomy is essential. This means that a good light is necessary, and occasionally an assistant.
4. Good surgical technique involves attention to haemostasis, restoration of normal anatomy, and the avoidance of excessive suturing.

4.5   STEPS IN EPISIOTOMY REPAIR

4.5.1   Step one

After analgesia is obtained, the vagina and perineum are carefully checked for any additional tears.

4.5.2   Step two

A suture of 441 chromic catgut is secured *above* the apex of the vaginal wound, leaving one end long. (Figure 4.3.)

4.5.3   Step three

The vaginal epithelium is repaired by continuous locked sutures down to the fourchette, taking particular care to match up the hymenal remnants (caruncules myrtiformes) at the introitus. This suture is then secured with a knot in the deep tissues. (Figure 4.5.)

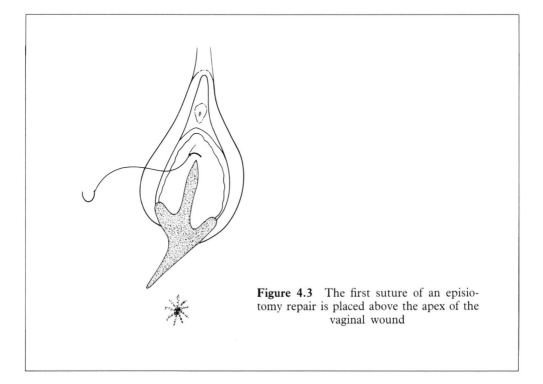

Figure 4.3 The first suture of an episiotomy repair is placed above the apex of the vaginal wound

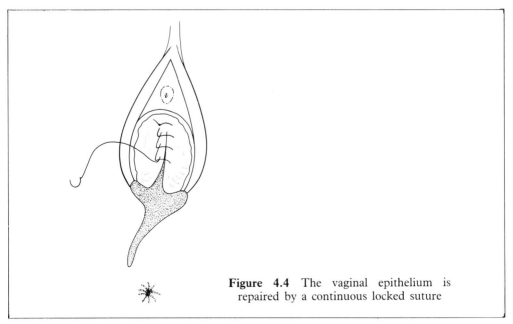

Figure 4.4 The vaginal epithelium is repaired by a continuous locked suture

4.5.4   Step four

The deep layers are repaired with interrupted sutures, taking care medially not to insert a suture through the rectal mucosa; 2/0 chromic catgut suture with a round bodied needle is appropriate for this part of the repair. Successively more superficial sutures are inserted so as to obliterate any dead space and achieve haemostasis. (Figure 4.6.)

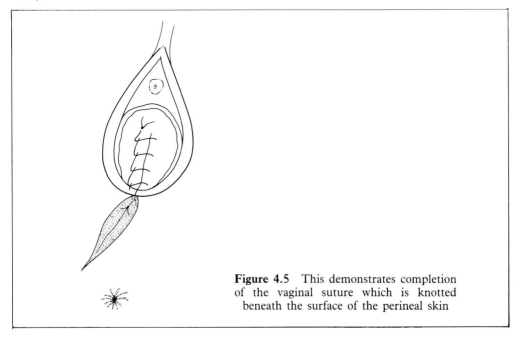

Figure 4.5 This demonstrates completion of the vaginal suture which is knotted beneath the surface of the perineal skin

4.5.5 Step five

When the skin edges are almost opposed the skin suture is inserted. The best results in terms of patient comfort and good healing are achieved with a subcuticular suture as shown (Figures 4.7 and 4.8). The end is either knotted on the outside of the skin, or knotted to a long end left from the starting point of the suture which can be trailed across the incision.

In the case of a perineal tear, where the skin margins are ragged, inverted sutures can be inserted as in Figures 4.9 and 4.10.

4.5.6 Step six

A vaginal examination is performed to check that there is no continued bleeding and no remaining lacerations.

4.5.7 Step seven

A rectal examination is performed to check that no sutures are palpable. If a suture has breached the rectal mucosa, the entire repair must be taken down because of the risk of fistula formation and re-done.

4.6 REPAIR OF TEARS

1. Firstly the vagina and perineum are examined to determine the extent of the tear(s).
2. Occasionally there are two parallel posterior vaginal tears. In these cases it is

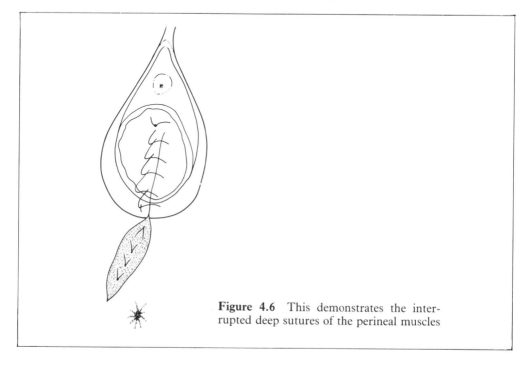

Figure 4.6 This demonstrates the interrupted deep sutures of the perineal muscles

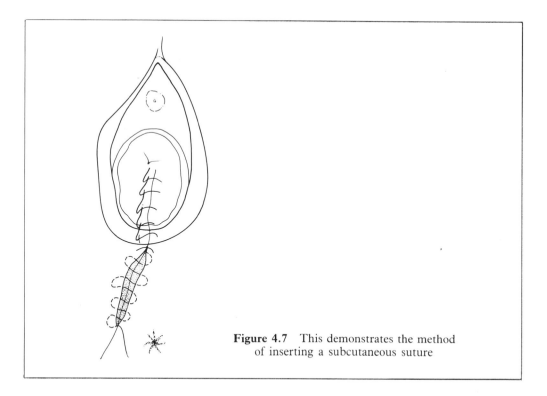

Figure 4.7   This demonstrates the method of inserting a subcutaneous suture

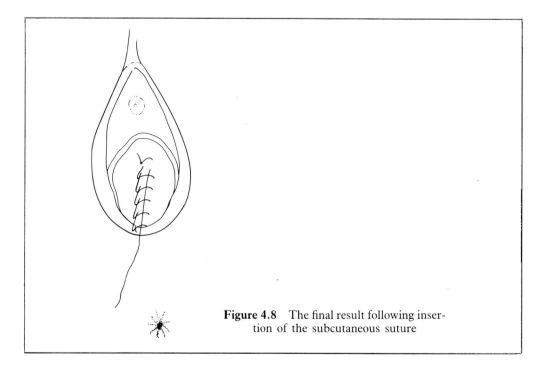

Figure 4.8   The final result following insertion of the subcutaneous suture

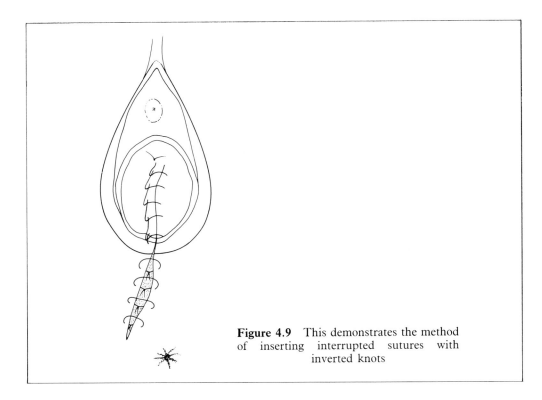

Figure 4.9 This demonstrates the method of inserting interrupted sutures with inverted knots

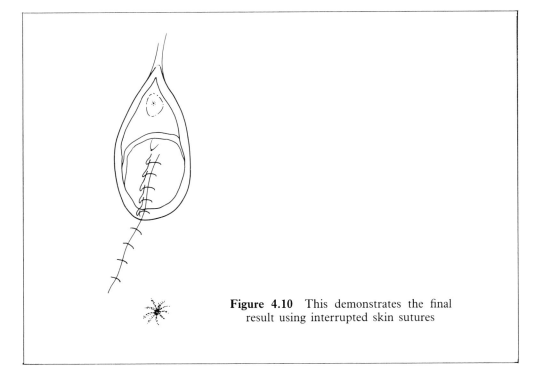

Figure 4.10 This demonstrates the final result using interrupted skin sutures

important to start to suture the vaginal epithelium on both sides at the same time, gradually working towards the introitus. If each tear is dealt with separately, it is difficult to get adequate access to the second tear, after the first has been completed.

3. Use 4/0 plain catgut interrupted sutures for the perineum and/or labia.
4. Superficial lacerations require no suturing, unless they are bleeding.
5. Lacerations in close proximity to the external urethral meatus are best repaired after insertion of a urethral catheter. This will identify the urethra and enable the operator to avoid inserting a suture into the urethra. It is probably advisable to leave the catheter *in situ* if it is felt that there is a reasonable risk of acute urinary retention secondary to local discomfort after the procedure. It could then be removed after 24–48 h.
6. See Chapter 25 for repair of a third degree tear or a cervical tear.

Chapter 5
The Puerperium

5.1 INTRODUCTION

The puerperium is a time of adaptation to a new situation during which the recently delivered mother requires informed advice and support. It is a time during which physiological processes may rapidly revert to the non-pregnant state. Some of these will occur earlier than others; some will take several months to be complete. A knowledge of this timing is important when considering investigations after delivery, e.g. investigation of the upper urinary tract is best deferred until at least three months postpartum.

The puerperium is also a time of psychological changes. Insecurity, apprehension and anxiety are often felt by the new mother. Very rarely frank psychotic reactions may also occur. The length of hospital stay after delivery will obviously depend upon the wishes of the mother, the help available at home, the mode of delivery, whether any complications occurred, and upon the hospital bed availability. An increasing number of women are discharged after a very short time (6–48 h).

The average length of hospital stay is four to seven days. The disadvantage of early discharge is that complications may occur at home where the woman has no easy access to medical or midwifery attention. In these situations it is important to ensure that there is adequate support at home, and that community services will be provided.

5.2 UNCOMPLICATED PUERPERIUM

5.2.1 Breast and bottle feeding

Most women will have attended antenatal classes and will have been instructed in the relative benefits of each method. The choice should be left to the mother. Women who do not choose to breast feed or in whom breastfeeding is to be discontinued should be given no treatment other than a firm supporting maternity brassiere. If engorgement develops, one or two tablets of paracetamol (1 g) every 4 h are usually sufficient for pain relief until lactation subsides.

In women with persistent lactation or in those who had a stillbirth or neonatal death 2.5 mg of bromocriptine should be given on day one followed by 2.5 mg twice a day for fourteen days.

5.2.2 Routine investigations

Blood should be sent for haemoglobin estimation on the second day postpartum. Any woman catheterized during or after labour should have a mid-stream specimen of urine (MSU) collected the same day and sent for microscopy, culture and sensitivity.

5.2.3 Episiotomy care

Discomfort from an episiotomy repair or laceration can be relieved by simple analgesics such as paracetamol, or the application of an ice pack. Frequent bathing with saline or use of a bidet will encourage healing and antisepsis, and the area can be dried effectively with an electric hair-dryer. Occasionally a superficial dehiscence of the episiotomy margins may occur, but it is very unusual for secondary re-suturing to be necessary.

5.2.4 Prevention of Rhesus iso-immunization

100 µg (500 i.u.) of Anti-D is given intramuscularly to all Rhesus negative women delivered of Rhesus positive infants, within 72 h of delivery, after the result of cord blood grouping. A Kleihauer test is performed on all Rhesus negative women after delivery. This detects the extent of feto–maternal bleeding which inevitably occurs at the time of delivery. If there are 80 fetal red cells in 50 low power fields, this corresponds to a 4 ml feto–maternal bleed. If the maternal Kleihauer test suggests that a feto–maternal haemorrhage in excess of 4 ml has occurred, then the haematology department may advise an additional dose of 100 µg Anti-D to be given to the mother. If for any reason the cord grouping is not known, then Anti-D should be given.

5.2.5   Rubella vaccination

Those women who have been found to be susceptible to rubella by antenatal serology should be offered vaccination in the puerperium, on the understanding that effective contraception is required for the next three months. This is preferably by means of a reliable method such as oral contraception or depot progestogen injections. It is usual to confirm immunity after vaccination prior to a further pregnancy.

5.2.6   Contraception and sterilization

It is important to discuss contraception with every woman in the puerperium as this is an ideal opportunity for education and advice. This can be done by the family planning nurse, family-planning-trained midwife or SHO.

Women who are given bromocriptine for suppression of lactation in particular may ovulate very early and should be warned that their fertility may return rapidly. Many women defer sexual intercourse until after their postnatal examination at six weeks, but there is usually no medical reason why this should be necessary, provided they understand that contraception should be used even if they are breast feeding.

The available alternatives are:

1. Progesterone-only pill (POP)
    This is a commonly used form of contraception by women who wish to breast feed. Combined pills carry a theoretical risk of suppression of milk production and the hazards of thromboembolism. The POP should be taken at the same time every day, and can be commenced on the tenth day after delivery. Protection should not be assumed until two weeks later.
2. Combined oral contraceptive pill.
    This may be commenced on the fourteenth day after delivery, by which time the hypercoagulable state of pregnancy has reverted to normal. Protection from pregnancy is immediate.
3. Sterilization.
    Sterilization during the course of a Caesarean section or in the early puerperium should not be undertaken lightly for the following reasons:
    a. It carries a greater risk to the woman of thromboembolic complications.
    b. It carries a greater risk of failure.
    c. It is preferable to ensure as far as possible the health of the newborn before embarking on such a permanent method of contraception.
    d. Laparoscopic sterilization as an interval procedure can be carried out with the minimum of social disruption, on a day-patient basis, at three months.

The request for sterilization should not be used as an argument for Caesarean section. The procedure, its risks and particularly the risk of failure, should be discussed and recorded in writing in the notes and on the operation consent form before being undertaken.

4. Depot-progestogens, e.g. Medroxy-progesterone acetate (MPA) 150 mg by deep
    intramuscular injection.
        This drug is licensed by the Committee on Safety of Medicines for use in two
    specific instances:
    a. To cover the three-month period after a woman has been given the Rubella
        vaccine
    b. To cover the period following vasectomy until sperm clearance.
        It provides contraception for three months. Its main disadvantages are the high
    incidence of irregular vaginal bleeding, and the fact that it is irreversible
    during that time. For this reason it tends to be used as a last resort where other
    methods have failed or are unsuitable.
5. Intra-uterine Contraceptive Device (IUCD).
    This can be inserted at the six-week postnatal examination if the woman requests
    it.

5.3   COMPLICATED PUERPERIUM

5.3.1   Superficial thrombophlebitis

This is an inflammatory (not infective) phenomenon where a clot forms in a superficial
vein of the leg leading to a localized tender, red swelling over the vein. Most cases will
settle spontaneously.
    Management:

1. Rest.
2. Support ('Tubigrip').
3. Analgesia.
4. Anti-inflammatory agent e.g. paracetamol.
5. Glycerine and icthyol poultice.

5.3.2   Deep venous thrombosis

Thrombo-embolic complications such as deep venous thrombosis or pulmonary
embolism (see Section 16.6) are more likely to occur in labour or the immediate
puerperium.
    Early diagnosis and appropriate treatment is essential for the health of the patient,
and because of the implications for future pregnancies (Section 16.6).

5.3.2.1   ASSOCIATED RISK FACTORS

1. Infection.
2. Operative delivery.
3. Trauma.
4. Obesity.

5. Advancing maternal age and parity.
6. High dose oestrogen therapy (e.g. stilboestrol, formerly used for suppression of lactation).
7. Smoking.
8. Varicose veins.
9. A past history.

5.3.2.2 SIGNS AND SYMPTOMS

1. Painful tender calf or leg with difficulty in walking.
2. Swelling and redness.
3. Pyrexia.
4. Positive Homan's sign (this, however, is unreliable).

5.3.2.3 DIAGNOSIS

1. Clinically—difficult as signs and symptoms are rarely clear cut. Measurement of calf or upper leg circumference at fixed points may demonstrate that one leg is swollen.
2. Doppler ultrasound, using a simple Sonicaid device.
3. Venography—will detect 90–95 per cent of thrombi.
4. Radioactive iodine-labelled fibrinogen (not suitable if the woman is breast-feeding).

5.3.2.4 PREVENTION

1. Early mobilization.
2. Use of support tights or 'TED' stockings in women with varicose veins. These should be fitted after the patient has been measured properly. Poorly fitting stockings may do more harm than good.
3. Avoid the use of high dose oestrogens in the puerperium.
4. Consider the use of prophylactic low-dose sub-cutaneous heparin in 'at risk' women (see above) to cover labour and the puerperium.

5.3.2.5 TREATMENT

Full heparinization is necessary (40 000 units per 24 h) by intravenous infusion using a syringe pump for five to seven days followed by warfarin therapy for three months. (Breast feeding is possible on warfarin therapy, but not with Dindevan.) Bedrest is advised initially but when the leg is no longer tender, mobilization and physiotherapy are encouraged.

5.3.3 Puerperal infection

This is defined as a temperature of over 37.5 °C on two occasions more than 4 h apart. All such women should be carefully examined with particular reference to breasts, chest, abdomen, lochia and legs. A high vaginal swab, cervical swab, MSU and throat swab should be sent for culture unless there is an obvious source for the pyrexia. If the temperature exceeds 38 °C a blood culture must also be sent. Whilst awaiting the results it may be advisable to treat the woman with broad spectrum antibiotics such as Metronidazole (400 mg t.d.s. orally) and a cephalosporin e.g. Cephradine (250 mg q.d.s. orally).

If the pyrexia is thought to be due to mastitis, milk should be sent for culture and treatment with Flucoxacillin should be started as soon as the clinical diagnosis is made. The diagnosis is usually made by finding a warm hard red area within the affected breast. Treatment with antibiotics at this early stage is not contraindicated as it may well prevent the development of a breast abscess. Breast feeding should continue as it is very unlikely that the infected milk will affect the baby. If it is too tender to breast feed then the affected breast should be emptied with a breast pump until the tenderness subsides. If a breast abscess occurs, it will require surgical drainage.

5.3.4 Secondary postpartum haemorrhage

This is defined as bleeding from the genital tract in excess of 500 ml after the first 24 h after delivery.

The usual cause for this is retained placental fragments. Haemorrhage may be profuse and the first step is to resuscitate the patient by replacement of the intravascular volume.

5.3.4.1 MANAGEMENT

1. A 16 g intravenous cannula is inserted and fluid replacement is commenced, according to the patient condition.
2. At the same time blood is taken for haemoglobin estimation and cross-matching of two units of blood.
3. Antibiotic treatment is advisable, since low-grade infection is common.
4. Evacuation of the uterus is undertaken when placental fragments remain, and is performed by an *experienced* operator, since the risk of uterine perforation and over-curettage leading to Asherman's syndrome of amenorrhoea due to intra-uterine adhesions are greatest at this time.

5.3.5 Puerperal psychosis

It is common and natural for women to feel emotionally labile for 24–48 h, some four to five days after delivery. This may be prolonged by physical discomfort, anaesthesia, infection, operative delivery or physical exhaustion.

When psychosis occurs, it generally appears at seven to 21 days after delivery and midwifery and medical staff should be alert to the following possible signs of psychosis:

1. Confusion.
2. Delirium.
3. Disordered sleep.

4.   Hallucinations.
5.   Mania.
6.   Delusions.
7.   Morbid feelings.
8.   Inappropriate anxieties.

It is essential to exclude a physical cause such as infection for an acute confusional state. Immediate treatment for confusion or delerium should be 10 mg haloperidol by intramuscular injection.

A psychiatric opinion should be sought early on, and if at all possible mother and baby should be kept together. Specific mother and baby units for this purpose are available in some psychiatric hospitals, where the patient and her baby can remain together, but under constant surveillance.

There is a 20 per cent recurrence risk of a puerperal psychosis in future pregnancies, and it is recommended that at least two years elapse before a subsequent pregnancy.

Chapter 6

Neonatal Resuscitation

6.1   INTRODUCTION

Neonatal resuscitation must be carried out early and efficiently to give the newborn the best possible outlook. About 1 per cent of babies will require neonatal resuscitation and 40 per cent of those will be unexpected from the antenatal and intrapartum course. For this reason, all labour ward staff should be competent in providing basic resuscitation. Appendix II indicates the situations in which a paediatrician should be called prior to delivery.

6.2   EQUIPMENT

A purpose-built resuscitation trolley (Resuscitaire), should ideally be available in every delivery room. This consists of an overhead heater, an angled platform, suction apparatus and an oxygen supply with a bag and mask. Two straight bladed neonatal laryngoscopes should be available on each Resuscitaire.

6.3   PREPARING THE EQUIPMENT

A midwife should check all equipment daily as a routine and after each delivery. The paediatrician or person trained in resuscitation should arrive prior to each high risk delivery and re-check the equipment.

6.3.1   Method

1. Switch on overhead heater to warm towels on shelf.
2. Check laryngoscope bulb and battery.
3. Open the packet of an endotracheal tube of appropriate size (see Section 6.4.3) if no assistant is available. Check that appropriate connector is available.
4. Check the oxygen cylinder is full, or if from a wall supply that it is connected properly.
5. Check that the manometer is working.
6. Check that the bag and mask are working.
7. Check that suction catheters size 6, 8 and 10 FG are present.
8. Check that syringes, drugs and i.v. solutions which may be required are present. These include:
    a. Naloxone
    b. 4.2 per cent sodium bicarbonate
    c. 10 per cent dextrose
    d. 10 per cent calcium gluconate
    e. 1 in 10 000 adrenaline
9. Reset the clock/timer.

6.4   ASSESSMENT AND IMMEDIATE MANAGEMENT

Successful transition to postnatal life depends on the establishment of:

1. Efficient respiration.
2. Efficient cardiac output.

6.4.1   When resuscitation is not necessary

Any baby who is likely to be asphyxiated should be transferred to the Resuscitaire and the clock started. The baby should be rapidly dried to prevent evaporative heat loss and then should be wrapped in warm dry towels.

An assessment of the baby's colour, respiration, heart rate and tone will contribute to an Apgar score being calculated at the end of the first minute (see Table 6.1). This provides a basis for subsequent management.

If the baby is breathing well, and the heart rate is greater than 100 beats min^{-1} and has a good colour he can be handed back to his mother.

6.4.2   When resuscitation is necessary

Apgar score 0–6.

Table 6.1 Apgar scores

Score	2	1	0
Parameter			
1. Heart rate	>100 beats min^{-1}	<100 beats min^{-1}	Absent
2. Respiratory effort	Crying	Slow	Absent
3. Muscle tone	Good	Some flexion of extremities	Flaccid
4. Reflex irritability	Cough, cry	Grimace	Absent
5. Colour	All pink	Trunk pink	Blue or white

Babies with scores of 0–2 are severely asphyxiated and are sometimes described as suffering from terminal or secondary apnoea, whilst babies with scores of 3–6 are described as suffering from primary apnoea.

6.4.3 Method of resuscitation

1. The mouth should be gently aspirated, followed by the nose, using a suction catheter. Excessive posterior pharyngeal suction must be avoided as it causes bradycardia by a vagal reflex.
2. If there has been meconium-staining of the liquor, aspiration of the trachea below the vocal cords should be carried out under laryngoscopic vision. If possible this should be before the first breath, to prevent meconium-aspiration but in practice the baby frequently gasps before this procedure can be effectively performed.
3. An appropriately-sized face mask and anaesthetic bag with oxygen supply can then be applied to the baby's face and the lungs gently inflated. The infant will usually improve in colour and commence spontaneous respiration.
4. If no such improvement is observed, after 1 min and the heart rate remains less than 50 beats min^{-1}, intubation and external cardiac massage are necessary.

    The laryngoscope blade is inserted into the right side of the baby's mouth towards the oropharynx. The baby's neck is slightly extended, to enable clear visualization of the cords by the operator. Over-extension of the baby's neck will result in difficult intubation. If necessary, light external pressure on the larynx will bring the cords into view (Figure 6.1). A 2.5 mm endotracheal tube is appropriate for very low birth weight babies (i.e. <1500 g or about 32 weeks) 3.0 mm for 32–37 week infants and 3.5 mm for full-term infants.

    The endotracheal tube is advanced along the blade of the laryngoscope, and through the glottis up to a distance of 2 cm. The smaller the baby, the shorter the distance the tube should be advanced through the cords.

    Give oxygen at a flow rate of less than 2 min^{-1}. For the first two breaths the inflation should be maintained for 2–3 s. After this 30–40 half second inflations should be given per minute.

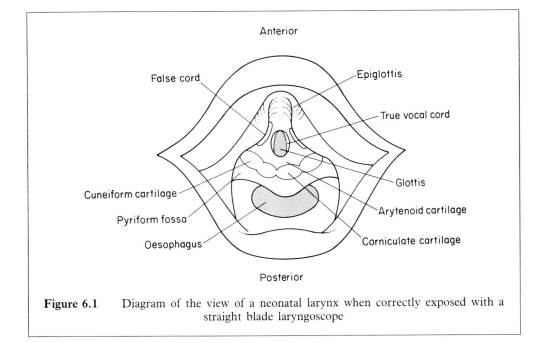

Figure 6.1   Diagram of the view of a neonatal larynx when correctly exposed with a straight blade laryngoscope

Auscultation over each side of the chest will check that air entry is equal. If the tube is in the right main bronchus with no air entry on the left, this is corrected by withdrawing the tube a little.

If the abdomen rises and falls, with no air entry in the chest, then the tube is in the oesophagus and re-intubation should be attempted.

If the air entry is diminished, but equal on each side, a suction catheter should be passed through the tube to exclude obstruction. If this fails to improve air entry, re-intubation should be attempted.

The endotracheal tube should be left *in situ* for a further 2 min after spontaneous breathing has become established.

6.4.4   External cardiac massage

External cardiac massage should be given if the heart rate is less than 50 beats min^{-1} in spite of good respiration. This is done by compression of the heart between the sternum and spine by the operator's thumb and fingers. Eight beats are given initially followed by four beats for each lung inflation. Cardiac output is checked by palpating femoral pulses.

1. If there is still no improvement in the baby's condition, drug therapy must be considered.
   a. Sodium bicarbonate 5 ml 8.4 per cent diluted with 50/50 10 per cent dextrose should be injected slowly via the umbilical vein.

    b.   If it is likely that respiratory depression is due to maternal narcotic analgesia, Naloxone, a specific and safe antagonist, can be given. The dose is 0.5–1.0 ml for preterm infants and 1.0–2.0 ml for full term infants.

    c.   Adrenaline (0.5 ml of 1 in 10 000) can be given directly down the endotracheal tube if the profound bradycardia persists. This should be repeated as an intracardiac injection if necessary.

2.   If resuscitation is unsuccessful after 20 min with no effective cardiac output, irreversible cerebral damage is likely and it is appropriate to stop.

If the baby has suffered severe asphyxia, he should be transferred to the special care unit once his condition is stable, but the parents should be allowed a brief cuddle before he is taken away. The infant who has suffered only mild asphyxia should be returned to the parents as soon as possible, and in all instances a full explanation of the resuscitative measures necessary and the likelihood of further sequelae should be undertaken as soon as possible.

II

COMPLICATED LABOUR

A.   Obstetric Complications

Chapter 7

Induction of Labour

7.1 INTRODUCTION

Induction of labour is usually carried out when it is considered that awaiting the onset of spontaneous labour is more hazardous to the mother or the fetus than induction. All patients undergoing induction should therefore be considered as high risk and a constant labour attendant and continuous fetal heart rate monitoring is advised.

Induction of labour should be started early in the morning, that is before 0800 hours, such that if the induction fails a decision on future management can be made at the end of the working day.

7.2 ADMISSION PROCEDURE

Patients for induction should ideally be admitted the night before the procedure. The SHO should check the following:

1. That the indication for the induction still exists.
2. The gestational age, which ideally should have been confirmed by ultrasound examination in the first half of pregnancy.
3. That the presenting part is engaged.

If there are discrepancies the woman should be reviewed by the duty registrar and/ or a senior obstetrician before induction.

7.3   METHODS OF INDUCING LABOUR

The most common method of induction is by means of a prostaglandin pessary followed sometime later by artificial rupture of membranes (ARM) and a syntocinon infusion if necessary.

7.3.1   Prostaglandin pessaries

These are usually formulated as 3 mg of prostaglandin E_2.

7.3.1.1   METHOD

1. Having donned sterile disposable gloves a vaginal examination is performed and the Bishop's score is noted (Table 7.1). A 3 mg prostaglandin E_2 pessary is then lubricated with a little Hibitane cream and inserted into the posterior vaginal fornix. The procedure and the time that it was performed are then recorded in the notes.
2. External fetal heart rate monitoring should now be commenced. Some obstetricians will allow intermittent cardiotocographic (CTG) recordings as long as the tracing is reactive (demonstrates accelerations of the fetal heart rate) and there is no uterine activity; this should be recorded for 30 min. As soon as labour commences continuous CTG records are advised.
3. The vaginal examination is repeated 4 h later. If the fetal head is engaged an attempt should now be made to perform ARM. If ARM is impossible insert a further 3 mg prostaglandin E_2 pessary.

Table 7.1   The Bishop's score

Features	Score			
	0	1	2	3
Cervical dilatation (cm)	0	1–2	3–4	>5
Cervical consistency	Firm	Medium	Soft	
Length of cervical canal (cm)	>2	2–1	1–0.5	<0.5
Cervical position	Posterior	Central	Anterior	
Station of presenting part (cm above ischial spines)	3	2	1–0	Below

4. Start an infusion of syntocinon (see Section 7.3.3) if labour has not commenced 2 h after the ARM.
5. If a second prostaglandin pessary was necessary the patient should be examined 4 h later and a further attempt should be made to perform ARM. If this is still not possible the patient should be reviewed by a senior obstetrician to decide if:
   a. A Caesarean section should be performed for a failed induction.
   b. The induction should continue by means of a further prostaglandin pessary or by ARM performed after epidural analgesia.
   c. The procedure should be abandoned and restarted the next day. A word of caution is necessary about this practice as labour may commence insidiously whilst the patient is asleep putting the fetus at risk, especially if it is growth retarded. It is wise, therefore, to perform a CTG late at night and early the next morning if this practice is to be followed.

7.3.2 Artificial rupture of the membranes (ARM)

This is usually performed after labour has been induced by means of prostaglandin pessaries but may be performed in the first instance if the cervix is very favourable (more than 4 cm dilated).

7.3.2.1 METHOD

1. An abdominal palpation is performed to confirm the presentation and to ensure the presenting part is engaged.
2. A vaginal examination is performed with the usual antiseptic precautions.
3. The index finger and the middle finger of the examining hand are inserted into the cervix. An Amnihook (Figure 7.1) or a pair of Kocher's forceps is guided through the cervix between the two fingers. The membranes are ruptured either by a sharp upward motion of the Amnihook or by grasping the membranes in the Kocher's forceps and pulling. If the ARM is successful you will usually be rewarded with a gush of fluid, note its colour.
4. If amniotic fluid is not obtained either the membranes remain intact or there is little or no fluid present. Repeat the procedure, if a fetal hair is obtained with the Kocher's forceps the membranes must be ruptured. If amniotic fluid is not obtained after a second attempt with the Amnihook a fetal scalp electrode should be attached and if a clear fetal heart rate signal is obtained the membranes have been ruptured.
5. A fetal scalp electrode is applied and attached to a monitor by an assistant. The examiner's fingers should not be removed until a clear fetal heart rate signal is obtained. The electrode should be re-applied if necessary.
6. The woman's vulva is dried and a sanitary towel is applied. The patient is made comfortable and the procedure is recorded in the patient's notes.

7.3.3 Syntocinon

Syntocinon is a synthetic oxytocin that will stimulate uterine activity. It is most effective as a means of inducing labour when administered to a patient who has already had vaginal prostaglandins. As a general rule it should not be administered to patients with intact membranes because of the risk of amniotic fluid embolism (see Section 16.5).

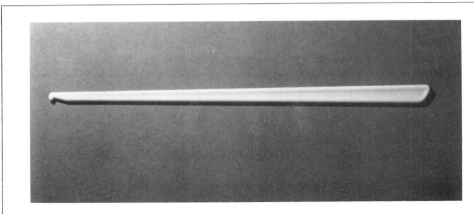

Figure 7.1   An amnihook

7.3.3.1   METHOD:

1. The infusion is made up by putting 10 iu of syntocinon in 1 l of Hartmann's solution. It should be infused by means of an infusion pump via a large bore (at least 16 gauge) cannula. In order to avoid the possibility of a bolus injection the infusion bag and giving set should *not* be attached to the cannula unless it already passes through the pump.
2. Start the infusion at *10 drops min*$^{-1}$ and increase it *every 30 min* in the following way:
    10 drops min^{-1} (5 mu min^{-1})
    20 drops min^{-1} (10 mu min^{-1})
    40 drops min^{-1} (20 mu min^{-1})
    60 drops min^{-1} (30 mu min^{-1})
    80 drops min^{-1} (40 mu min^{-1}).
    These mu equivalents are for standard giving sets where 20 drops of water are equivalent to 1 ml.
3. The infusion should be increased until the woman is contracting two to three times every 10 min. If at subsequent vaginal examination there is no progress as judged by cervical dilatation the infusion should be increased to 80 drops min^{-1} (40 mu min^{-1}) regardless of how frequently contractions occur. Subsequent vaginal examinations should be performed by the duty registrar as he/she will have to decide when to call a halt and perform a Caesarean section.
4. Fetal distress
    Should an abnormality of the CTG (Figure 15.7 for instance) occur during the course of the syntocinon infusion:
    a.   Stop the infusion.
    If the abnormality persists:
    b.   Turn the patient on her left side and give oxygen via a face mask at 4 l min^{-1}.
    c.   Perform a vaginal examination and a fetal blood sample (see Section 15.5).

d. If the fetal blood sample is normal (or in the absence of blood sampling facilities if the CTG returns to normal) restart the syntocinon 30 min later at half the preceeding rate. Repeat the fetal blood sample as indicated if the CTG remains abnormal. Although in many cases stopping the syntocinon will allow the fetal heart rate to return to normal, delivery will not occur in the absence of uterine activity so syntocinon must be administered.

e. If the fetal blood sample shows asphyxia then operative delivery is indicated.

7.3.3.2   CONTRAINDICATIONS TO SYNTOCINON REGIMEN

1. Grand multiparae (that is those with more than four previous births).
2. Patients with uterine scars.

These patients should have only 5 i.u. syntocinon to 1 ℓ of Hartmann's solution and the dose should be increased from 10 to 20 to 40 to 80 drops min^{-1}. If the patient is still not in labour or has dysfunctional labour the infusion strength should only be increased after the patient has been carefully reviewed. In these situations intra-uterine pressure monitors (see Section 7.4) may help.

7.4   INTRA-UTERINE PRESSURE MONITORING

This may be performed by means of:

1. A fluid-filled tube inserted into the uterus and connected to an external pressure transducer.
2. An intra-uterine catheter (Gaeltec) that has the pressure transducer mounted on its tip (Figure 7.2). These are sterilized by immersion into a solution of Cidex for 12 h. As they are solid they cannot block. They have a life of about 200 labours.

7.4.1   Insertion

The Gaeltec catheter is washed and then passed into the uterus, guided past the presenting part by the index and middle finger of the examiner's hand. The fluid-filled catheter is passed in a similar fashion and when amniotic fluid returns along the catheter the uterine cavity has been entered. It is then flushed with normal saline and attached to the transducer on the fetal heart rate monitor.

7.4.2   Interpretation of the results

1. Fluid-filled catheters. The external transducer should be set at the same height as where the tip is thought to lie. The baseline level is set such that the resting tone of the uterus is between 5–15 mmHg. The uterus may now be stimulated with syntocinon until the contractions have an amplitude of 60–70 mmHg. If no cervical dilatation occurs after 6 h at this level in a primipara or 3 h in a multipara a Caesarean section should be performed.

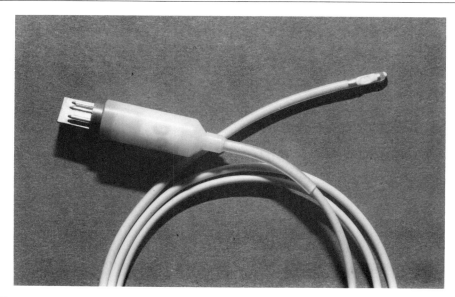

Figure 7.2   An intra-uterine pressure catheter (Gaeltec). The pressure transducer is mounted at the tip

    This catheter is also used to control the infusion rate in the Cardiff automatic infusion system (see below).
2. Gaeltec catheters. The machine is zeroed before the catheter is inserted by reference to a special storage and sterilizing tube supplied with the Gaeltec catheter. Once the transducer is inserted all transmission is electronic. Normal spontaneous labours have uterine activity levels of less than 1600 kPa per 15 min at 4 cm dilatation rising to 2400 kPa per 15 min at full dilatation. Stimulation with syntocinon up to these levels is therefore probably safe.

7.4.3   Possible indications

1. Premature rupture of membranes associated with failure to stimulate labour at 40 mu syntocinon min^{-1}.
2. Trial of scar (see Chapter 33).
3. Induction or augmentation in breech presentation.
4. Syntocinon augmentation in multigravid patients.

7.5   THE CARDIFF INFUSION SYSTEM

This is an attempt at providing automatic control of the syntocinon infusion based upon the frequency and amplitude of the induced uterine contractions. It has the following features:

1. A spring loaded drip stand that senses when the infusion bag is empty, switches the system off and sounds an alarm.
2. A rotary infusion pump. Ten units of syntocinon are placed in 500 ml of normal saline and connected through the infusion pump by means of a specially designed giving set that has a portion of narrow tubing of known calibre that passes around the rotary pump.
3. A pressure transducer for connection to a fluid-filled intra-uterine pressure catheter.
4. An automatic infusion system that is alarmed. The syntocinon infusion rate will double (to a maximum of 64 mu min^{-1}) as long as the contractions do not exceed 60 mmHg in amplitude and are not more frequent than one every 3 min. Values outside these limits or a rise in baseline tone will cause the system to stop and an alarm to sound.
5. The machine also detects fetal heart rate. It can be programmed to switch off and to sound an alarm if the heart rate is outside pre-set limits.
6. The infusion rate can also be increased manually by means of a dial.

7.6 COMPLICATIONS

The most common complication of induction of labour is a failed induction. The use of prostaglandin pessaries combined with ARM and syntocinon infusion (if necessary) results in a 5 per cent failure rate. This figure is as high as 30 per cent following ARM alone. Other complications are of the individual methods:

7.6.1 Prostaglandin pessaries

1. Pyrexia. About 1 per cent of all patients given prostaglandin pessaries will develop a mild pyrexia in labour, but does not generally exceed 37.5 °C and is not usually a clinical problem. Temperatures exceeding this value should be investigated (see Chapter 10).
2. Precipitate labour. Occasionally a grand multigravid patient will have a very rapid labour following insertion of a prostaglandin pessary. The pessary should be removed if possible. If fetal distress arises or the patient is unable to cope with the contractions they can be reduced in frequency by an infusion of ritodrine (see Section 9.6).

7.6.2 Syntocinon infusion

1. Fetal distress. This may be the result of hyperstimulation. The infusion should be stopped and the fetal heart rate observed over the next 10 min. If the abnormality of the CTG persists a fetal blood sample should be performed. If the CTG returns to normal and/or the fetal blood sample is normal the infusion should be recommenced after 30 min at half the preceeding rate.
2. Water intoxication. Syntocinon has antidiuretic hormone-like activity and so if administered in large amounts with salt-free solutions may result in severe hyponatraemia of both the mother and the neonate. This may be prevented by diluting syntocinon in normal saline and critically reviewing fluid balance in all patients who receive more than 3 ℓ of fluid in labour.

3. Amniotic fluid embolism. This complication of syntocinon administration only occurs if syntocinon is given to patients with intact membranes.
4. Ruptured uterus. This complication is almost unheard of in primiparous patients and only occurs with poor management in multiparous patients. Extra care should be taken in giving syntocinon to patients with uterine scars (see Chapter 33).

7.6.3   Artificial rupture of the membranes (ARM)

1. Prolapsed cord. This complication only occurs if the fetal head is not engaged when the membranes are ruptured or if there is an unrecognized cord presentation.
2. Fetal distress. A single, sometimes deep and profound deceleration of the fetal heart may occur immediately after ARM. This is thought to be due to a combination of fetal head compression and the effect of sudden decompression on placental function. The fetal heart rate usually returns to normal soon after. If not a fetal blood sample should be performed.
3. Prolonged rupture of the membranes. Once the membranes have been ruptured for more than 24 h there is an increased incidence of fetal distress probably due to declining placental function. The risk of chorioamnionitis is also said to be increased. Stopping syntocinon overnight in patients with ruptured membranes is therefore not a wise practice.

Chapter 8
Dysfunctional Labour

8.1 INTRODUCTION

Dysfunctional labour may lead to prolonged labour (dystocia) with the following risks:

1. Increased maternal anxiety. A long labour leads to increasing maternal anxiety with the consequent release of catecholamines. Noradrenaline causes abnormal uterine activity with contractions arising from the lower segment rather than the fundus. These contractions are more painful and do not cause cervical dilatation. This leads to a vicious circle being set up which is known as the pain-fear-anxiety syndrome.
2. Increasing maternal dehydration. Fluid loss in labour may be substantial because of hyperventilation and decreased maternal intake and unless fluid is replaced *ketosis* will occur. This is evidence of increasing maternal acidosis. The increase in hydrogen ion production in the maternal circulation inhibits uterine activity by competing with calcium. Thus dehydration leads to further delay in labour.
3. Loss of confidence in the attendants. Most women expect to deliver within 12–14 h from the onset of labour. If adequate explanation for the delay in labour is not provided and more particularly if the woman is left unattended she will rapidly lose confidence and become less co-operative.
4. Increased risk of fetal distress. Prolonged labour is associated with depletion of fetal reserves and a higher incidence of operative delivery for fetal distress.
5. Increased risk of infection. Prolonged rupture of the membranes increases the risk of chorioamnionitis with its increased incidence of fetal distress. If Caesarean section becomes necessary the risk of subsequent puerperal sepsis is increased by at least five-fold.

All the above complications increase the chances of operative delivery with its attendant complications. In view of this most obstetric units now practice some form of active management of labour. This involves the use of a partogram to summarize the progress of labour (see Section 1.4) and as an aid to the recognition of the abnormalities of labour.

8.2   ABNORMALITIES OF LABOUR

There are three recognized abnormalities of labour.

8.2.1   Prolonged latent phase (PLP)

The latent phase is defined as the time from the onset of labour to the point in time at which the cervix is full effaced. It is often only possible to recognize the latent phase retrospectively. Prolonged latent phase (PLP) is uncommon, occurring in less than 5 per cent of primigravidae and being very rare in multigravidae as the cervix effaces and dilates at the same time.

8.2.1.1   CAUSES

1. Idiopathic (most cases). In some patients no obvious cause is apparent but if the presenting part is high cervical ripening in late pregnancy may not occur.
2. Incorrect diagnosis of labour. False labour or pre-labour occurs when the woman complains of painful contractions but they have no effect on the cervix. The uterine activity usually subsides after a few hours. Interference by means of ARM however will often lead to PLP.
3. Premature rupture of the membranes (PROM). This term refers to rupture of the membranes occurring at term in the absence of uterine activity. Current management is to induce labour within 12 h by means of a syntocinon infusion. This often results in a PLP and up to 20 per cent of such patients will come to Caesarean section for failed induction.
4. Cervical dystocia. This term is used for a cervix that fails to dilate despite adequate uterine contractions and syntocinon augmentation. It is very rare but is usually associated with scarring due to previous cervical surgery, for example after cone biopsy or following a long-standing cervical suture. A few cases are idiopathic.

8.2.1.2   MANAGEMENT

Make a correct diagnosis of labour. The diagnosis of labour is usually made by observing progressive effacement and dilatation of the cervix with time. Patients who present with uterine contractions and who may or may not be in early labour should have no interference (aside from appropriate monitoring of the fetus) until the fetal head is fully engaged, the cervix is fully effaced and is at least 4 cm dilated. Adherence to this will largely avoid the problem of PLP.

The small group of women who have painful contractions in the presence of minimal cervical change should be given 15–20 mg of Omnopon im. This will cause uterine activity to cease in about half whilst those who were indeed in early labour will continue to labour but will be relatively pain free.

Very rarely, painful uterine contractions which cause cervical effacement but minimal dilatation will continue (Figure 8.1) and these women should be given syntocinon (see Section 7.3.3). This is one of the very few situations when it may be necessary to give syntocinon with intact membranes. Repeat the vaginal examination every 3 h. Rupture the membranes (if not already ruptured) as soon as possible.

8.2.1.3 OUTCOME

Most patients will go on to have a normal active phase of labour. About 15 per cent, however, will require a Caesarean section and this should be performed after there has been no progress with the syntocinon infusion at its maximum rate (40 mu min^{-1}) for 6 h.

8.2.2 Secondary arrest of cervical dilatation (SACD)

This occurs when the patient enters the active phase normally but then the cervix stops dilating, commonly at 5–6 cm. It occurs in about 5 per cent of primigravid and 2 per cent of multigravid women.

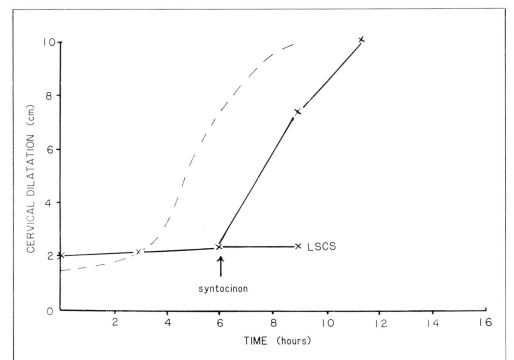

Figure 8.1 Prolonged latent phase. The dotted line indicates the line of expected progress. The patient's progress is marked by the solid line. The possible outcomes following the administration of syntocinon are indicated

8.2.2.1 CAUSE

1. Malposition and/or poor flexion of the fetal head. This is the commonest cause. The vaginal examination will commonly reveal poor flexion, the anterior fontanelle being directly beneath the examining fingers as they enter the cervix (see Figure 20.2).
2. Cephalo-pelvic disproportion. In this situation the vaginal examination usually demonstrates a well-flexed head with moulding.
3. Malpresentation.

Note: We have not included poor/inco-ordinate uterine activity as a cause for SACD because we believe that it is rarely a primary cause but is secondary to the obstruction.

8.2.2.2 MANAGEMENT

1. Perform a vaginal examination to exclude a malpresentation.
2. Start a syntocinon infusion as detailed in Section 7.3.3.
3. Repeat the vaginal examination every 3 h.

8.2.2.3 OUTCOME

Figure 8.2 illustrates the possible outcomes. About 75 per cent of patients will respond to the syntocinon infusion and come to a vaginal delivery. This seems to be due to the syntocinon stimulating good uterine contractions which cause flexion (and rotation) of the fetal head.

Those patients who fail to respond to syntocinon have a diagnosis of cephalopelvic disproportion and should undergo Caesarean section after 6 h of full dose (40 mu min^{-1}) syntocinon for primigravidae and 3 h in the case of a multigravidae. There is a very low incidence of fetal distress in this condition.

8.2.3 Primary dysfunctional labour (PDL)

This is the second abnormality of the active phase of labour and is said to occur when the rate of cervical dilatation in the active phase is less than 1 cm h^{-1}. It occurs in a quarter of all primigravid and about 10 per cent of multigravid labours. It has the worst prognosis of all with a higher incidence of Caesarean section and fetal distress.

8.2.3.1 CAUSE

1. Inefficient uterine action. These patients often demonstrate inco-ordinated uterine activity with coupled contractions and hypertonus. These contractions are not efficient, are more painful and cervical dilatation does not occur.
2. Cephalo-pelvic disproportion.
3. Occipito-posterior position.

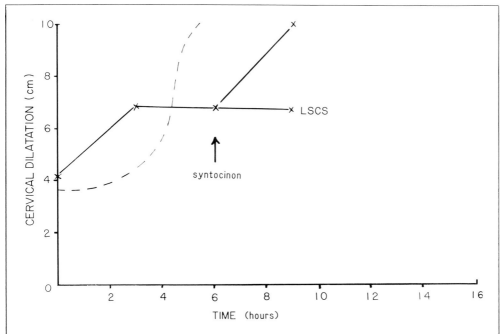

Figure 8.2   Secondary arrest of cervical dilatation. The possible outcomes following the administration of syntocinon are illustrated

8.2.3.2 MANAGEMENT

1. Perform a vaginal examination to exclude a malposition.
2. Rupture the membranes if they are intact and attach a fetal scalp electrode.
3. Start a syntocinon infusion as detailed in Section 7.3.3.
4. Provide adequate analgesia. As uterine activity in PDL is often inco-ordinate and especially if the position is occipito-posterior it is well worthwhile recommending epidural analgesia. This will provide a painless labour and will prevent the onset of the pain–fear–anxiety syndrome (see above).
5. Repeat the vaginal examination every 3 h.

8.2.3.3 OUTCOME

This is illustrated in Figure 8.3.

Giving a syntocinon infusion will improve the rate of cervical dilatation in over 80 per cent of women with PDL and most of these (all but about 5 per cent) will achieve a vaginal delivery.

Note: Patients with PDL who require forceps deliveries should be considered for a trial of forceps unless the head is very obviously in the pelvic outlet (see Chapter 26).

If syntocinon does not improve the rate of cervical dilatation 80 per cent of these women will come to delivery by Caesarean section. In most cases the reason for the

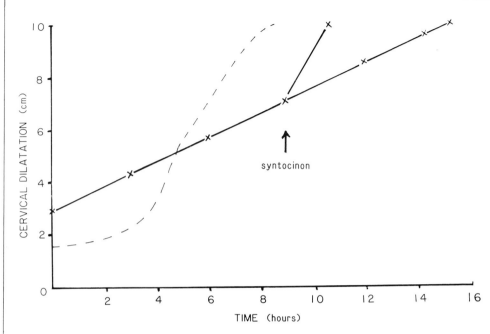

Figure 8.3   Primary dysfunctional labour. The possible outcomes following syntocinon administration are illustrated. Even if the rate of cervical dilatation improves Caesarean section is commonly necessary for fetal distress

Caesarean section will be fetal distress. Complete cessation of cervical dilatation in a multigravid patient despite full dose syntocinon should lead to Caesarean section because of the risks of uterine rupture.

8.3   MANAGEMENT AFTER DELIVERY

All women who have received syntocinon in labour are at high risk of a postpartum haemorrhage consequent on uterine atonia. This may be prevented by a prophylactic infusion of 40 i.u. of syntocinon in 500 ml of Hartmann's solution run at 80 drops min^{-1} for 2 h after delivery.

Chapter 9

Preterm Labour and Delivery

9.1   INTRODUCTION

Preterm labour is defined as labour occurring at less than 37 completed weeks of gestation. This occurs in about 6 per cent of the population but as the outlook for infants born between 34–37 weeks gestation is little different from those born at term the major problems occur with labour at less than 34 completed weeks of gestation. This accounts for about 2 per cent of the population but such infants contribute about 75 per cent of the perinatal mortality rate.

9.2 PROGNOSIS

The prognosis for preterm infants depends upon:

1. The availability of a neonatal intensive care unit (NICU). All infants born at less than 30 weeks gestation should, if time and maternal and fetal condition allow be transferred *in utero* to a hospital with a NICU. It may also be necessary to transfer women with older fetuses if local facilities could not care for such infants.
2. The gestational age and birthweight. Survival figures from your own hospital and the local regional NICU for different gestational ages should be known to help decide whether women should be transferred and to aid management. Table 9.1 illustrates survival figures from St George's hospital and has space for local figures.

Table 9.1 Approximate 28-day survival rates for preterm infants

Weeks	Weight (g)	Survival (%)	
		StG[a]	Local[b]
24	600	25	
25	750	35	
26	900	50	
28	1100	80	
30	1300	90	
32	1500	98	
>34	>2200	98	

[a] StG St George's Hospital
[b] Complete this with data for your own hospital

3. The condition of the baby at birth. Asphyxiated preterm infants have a much higher incidence and are more likely to die from respiratory distress syndrome (RDS). They also have an increased incidence of intraventricular haemorrhage (IVH). Continuous electronic fetal heart rate monitoring with frequent fetal blood samples for *any* abnormality of the heart rate is therefore mandatory.
4. Immediate neonatal management. Figure 9.1 illustrates the avoidable factors that lead to surfactant deficiency. A skilled neonatal team must therefore be present at the delivery to avoid factors such as hypothermia and postnatal asphyxia (see also Chapter 6).
5. The use of steroids to mature the lungs of fetuses of less than 32 weeks gestation. This is controversial and local practice must be known.

9.3 LOWER LIMITS OF PRETERM DELIVERY

The decision as to when one should actively monitor a preterm fetus at the lower limits of fetal viability should be agreed within each hospital. Approximately 10–25 per cent of infants born at 24 weeks gestation can be expected to survive with NICU facilities.

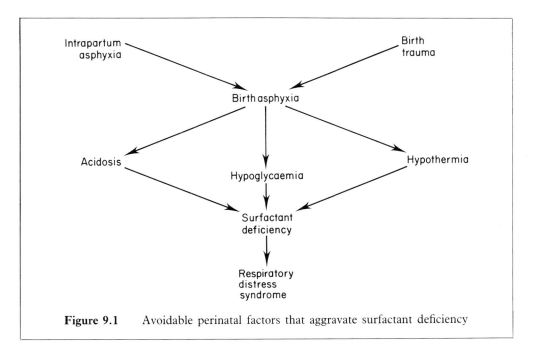

Figure 9.1   Avoidable perinatal factors that aggravate surfactant deficiency

Most hospitals will transfer women of this gestation to a regional NICU but obviously the decision has to be individualized.

Women who miscarry at whatever gestation feel a great sense of loss. They need sympathetic handling by skilled people (see Chapter 34). The maternity team is often the most appropriately trained to care for these women. It may therefore be entirely appropriate to manage the woman with a miscarriage at 18–24 weeks on the labour ward rather than the gynaecology wards.

9.4   DIAGNOSIS OF PRETERM LABOUR

Up to half of all women who present with painful contractions before 37 weeks gestation will stop spontaneously. On the other hand preterm labour may be insidious and result in the unexpected delivery of an unmonitored infant that is asphyxiated.

9.4.1   Procedure

1. All women in threatened preterm labour should have their antenatal history reviewed and a history of the recent events recorded. A physical examination should be performed looking for a cause (see Table 9.2).
2. If there is no history of ruptured membranes a vaginal examination should be performed using a sterile disposable glove and Hibitane cream. The findings should be recorded as illustrated in Table 1.1 but particular attention should be paid to the degree of effacement and dilatation.

Table 9.2   Causes of preterm labour

---

1. Preterm, premature rupture of the membranes

2. Cervical incompetence

3. Multiple pregnancy

4. Polyhydramnios

5. Antepartum haemorrhage

6. Fetal death

7. Maternal pyrexia

8. Uterine abnormalities

---

3. Management of patients with suspected rupture of the membranes is detailed in Chapter 10.

4. The fetal heart rate and uterine activity should be continuously recorded.

5. If two or more contractions are recorded every 10 min then the patient should have a repeat vaginal examination 2 h later by the same examiner. A change in the cervical effacement or dilatation confirms the diagnosis of labour.

9.5   PRINCIPLES OF MANAGEMENT

1. All labours occurring at less than 37 weeks gestation should be continuously monitored by electronic means. This allows the early detection of antenatal asphyxia which is one of the major factors determining the prognosis of the preterm infant (see Figure 9.1). Interpretation of the CTG patterns is the same as for term labour (see Section 15.4) but earlier recourse should be made to fetal blood sampling which should also be repeated more frequently if the CTG remains abnormal. Fetal blood sampling on preterm infants should be performed by the obstetric registrar. Interpretation of the results is found in Section 15.5

2. In women who present in suspected preterm labour a plan of management should be decided upon by the most senior obstetrician available in conjunction with the paediatric team. If *in utero* transfer is appropriate it should be arranged.

3. Management is aimed at delaying delivery for at least 48 hours so that steroid therapy may be effective in maturing the fetal lungs. This is controversial and the policy of the consultant on call should be consulted. Tocolysis (suppression of uterine activity) is also indicated to allow *in utero* transfer.

4. If there is doubt about the woman's gestation a fetal weight estimate should be obtained by ultrasound. The biparietal diameter (Figure 9.2) and the abdominal circumference (Figure 9.3) should be measured and the weight should be estimated from Table 9.3. Major fetal abnormalities should also be detected at this time.

5. Analgesia. Preterm infants metabolize drugs poorly so epidural analgesia is advised for all preterm labours. However, if the mother does not want epidural analgesia

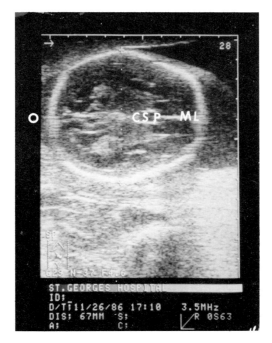

Figure 9.2   An ultrasound scan of a transverse section of fetal head at the correct level at which the biparietal diameter (+. . .+) is measured. (CSP = cavum septum pellucidum, O = occiput, ML = midline)

or it is not available, pethidine should be given in sufficient doses to control her pain. Sedatives have no role in uncomplicated preterm labour.

6.   Presentation. Breech and abnormal presentations at less than 32 weeks gestation should probably be delivered by Caesarean section (see below).

9.6   TOCOLYSIS

There is no convincing statistical evidence that tocolytic agents usefully prolong pregnancy. However, in women in whom the cervix is less than 4 cm dilated on admission delivery may often be delayed for 48 h to allow the steroids time to act.

9.6.1   Contraindications to tocolysis

These include situations where delay in delivery or the drugs used to delay delivery may be hazardous to the mother or the fetus.

Table 9.3   Chart of estimated fetal weights derived from the BPD and AC measurements. Reproduced by permission of McGraw-Hill

Abdominal circumference (mm)

BPD (mm)	40	45	50	55	60	65	70	75	80	85	90	95	100	105	110	115	120	125	130	135	140	145	150
30	80	83	87	91	95	99	104	108	113	118	123	129	135	141	147	154	161						
31	83	86	90	94	98	103	107	112	117	122	128	133	139	145	152	159	166	173	181				
32			93	97	102	106	111	116	121	126	132	138	144	150	157	164	171	178	186				
33			97	101	105	110	115	120	125	130	136	142	148	155	162	169	176	184	192				
34			100	104	109	114	119	124	129	135	141	147	153	160	167	174	182	190	198	206	215		
35					113	118	123	129	134	139	145	152	158	165	172	180	187	195	204	213	222		
36					117	122	127	134	138	144	150	157	163	170	176	183	193	202	210	219	229		
37					121	126	131	138	143	149	155	162	169	176	183	191	199	208	217	226	235	245	256
38							136	143	148	154	160	167	174	182	189	197	206	214	223	233	243	253	263
39							141	148	153	159	166	173	180	187	195	203	212	221	230	240	250	260	271

BPD (mm)	70	75	80	85	90	95	100	105	110	115	120	125	130	135	140	145	150	155	160	165	170	175	180
40	145	152	158	164	171	178	186	193	202	210	219	228	237	247	257	268	279						
41			163	170	177	184	192	200	208	217	226	235	245	255	265	276	288	299	312				
42			169	176	183	190	198	206	215	223	233	242	252	262	273	284	296	308	321				
43			174	182	189	197	205	213	222	231	240	250	260	270	281	293	305	317	330				
44			180	188	195	203	211	220	229	238	247	257	268	279	290	302	314	326	340	353	368		
45					202	210	218	227	236	245	255	265	276	287	299	311	323	336	349	363	378		
46					208	217	225	234	244	253	263	274	285	296	308	320	333	346	359	374	389		
47					215	224	233	242	251	261	271	282	293	305	317	329	342	356	370	384	400	415	432
48							240	250	259	269	280	291	302	314	326	339	352	366	381	395	411	427	444
49							248	258	268	278	289	300	312	324	336	349	363	377	392	407	422	439	456

BPD (mm)	100	105	110	115	120	125	130	135	140	145	150	155	160	165	170	175	180	185	190	195	200	205	210	215	220
50	256	266	276	287	298	309	321	334	346	360	374	388	403	418	434	451	468	486	505						
51			285	296	307	319	331	344	357	370	385	399	414	430	447	464	481	500	519						
52			294	305	317	329	341	354	368	381	396	411	426	443	459	477	495	513	533						
53			304	315	327	339	352	365	379	393	408	423	439	455	472	490	508	527	547	568	589				
54			315	327	337	350	363	376	390	405	420	435	451	468	486	504	522	542	562	583	605				
55					348	360	374	388	402	417	432	448	464	482	499	518	537	557	577	598	620				
56					359	372	385	399	414	429	445	461	478	495	513	532	552	572	593	614	637	660	684		
57							397	412	426	442	458	474	492	509	528	547	567	587	609	631	654	677	702		
58							409	424	439	455	471	488	506	524	543	562	583	604	625	648	671	695	720		
59									453	469	485	503	520	539	558	578	599	620	642	665	689	713	739	765	792

BPD (mm)	140	145	150	155	160	165	170	175	180	185	190	195	200	205	210	215	220	225	230	235	240	245	250
60	466	483	500	517	536	554	574	594	615	637	659	683	707	732	758	784	812						
61	480	497	514	532	551	570	590	611	632	654	677	701	725	751	777	804	832						
62			530	548	567	587	607	628	650	672	696	720	745	770	797	825	853	883	913				

	170	175	180	185	190	195	200	205	210	215	220	225	230	235	240	245	250	255	260	265	270	275	280	285	290
63	545	564	583	603	624	645	668	691	714	739	764	790	818	846	875	905	936								
64	561	580	600	621	642	664	686	709	734	759	784	811	839	867	897	927	959								
65	617	638	660	682	705	729	753	779	805	832	860	889	919	950	982	1015	1050								
66	635	657	678	701	725	749	774	800	826	854	882	912	942	974	1006	1040	1075								
67	654	675	698	721	745	769	795	821	848	876	905	935	966	998	1031	1065	1100	1137	1174						
68			717	741	765	790	816	843	870	899	928	959	990	1023	1056	1091	1127	1164	1202						
69			738	762	786	812	838	865	893	922	952	983	1015	1048	1082	1117	1154	1191	1230						
70	758	783	808	834	861	888	917	946	977	1008	1041	1074	1109	1144	1181	1219	1258	1299	1340						
71			830	857	884	912	941	971	1002	1034	1067	1101	1136	1172	1209	1248	1287	1328	1371						
72			853	880	908	936	966	996	1028	1060	1094	1128	1164	1200	1238	1277	1317	1359	1402						
73					932	961	991	1022	1054	1087	1121	1156	1192	1229	1268	1307	1348	1390	1433	1478	1524				
74					958	987	1018	1049	1081	1115	1149	1185	1221	1259	1298	1338	1379	1422	1466	1511	1558				
75					983	1013	1044	1076	1109	1143	1178	1214	1251	1290	1329	1370	1411	1455	1499	1545	1592	1641	1691		
76							1072	1104	1138	1172	1208	1244	1282	1321	1361	1402	1444	1488	1533	1579	1627	1676	1727		
77							1100	1133	1167	1202	1238	1275	1313	1353	1393	1435	1478	1522	1568	1615	1663	1713	1764		
78							1129	1163	1197	1233	1269	1307	1346	1385	1426	1469	1512	1557	1603	1651	1700	1750	1802	1855	1910
79									1228	1264	1301	1339	1379	1419	1461	1503	1547	1593	1639	1688	1737	1788	1840	1894	1950

	255	260	265	270	275	280	285	290	295	300	305	310	315	320	325	330	335	340	345	350	355	360	365	370	375
80	1260	1296	1334	1373	1412	1453	1495	1539	1583	1629	1677	1725	1775	1827	1880	1934	1990								
81			1367	1407	1447	1488	1531	1575	1620	1667	1715	1764	1814	1866	1920	1975	2032	2090	2150						
82			1402	1441	1482	1524	1568	1612	1658	1705	1753	1803	1854	1907	1961	2017	2074	2133	2193						
83			1437	1477	1519	1561	1605	1650	1697	1744	1793	1843	1895	1948	2003	2059	2117	2176	2237	2300	2365				
84					1556	1599	1643	1689	1736	1784	1834	1885	1937	1991	2046	2103	2161	2221	2282	2346	2411				
85					1594	1638	1683	1729	1776	1825	1875	1927	1979	2034	2090	2147	2206	2266	2328	2392	2458				
86							1723	1770	1818	1867	1918	1970	2023	2078	2134	2192	2252	2313	2375	2440	2506	2574	2644		
87							1764	1811	1860	1910	1961	2014	2068	2123	2180	2238	2298	2360	2423	2488	2555	2623	2694		
88							1806	1854	1903	1954	2005	2059	2113	2169	2227	2286	2346	2408	2472	2538	2605	2674	2745	2817	2892
89									1947	1998	2051	2104	2160	2216	2274	2334	2395	2457	2522	2588	2656	2725	2797	2870	2945
90	2044	2097	2151	2207	2264	2323	2383	2445	2508	2573	2639	2707	2778	2849	2923	2999									
91		2145	2199	2256	2313	2372	2433	2495	2559	2624	2692	2760	2831	2903	2977	3054	3132	3212							
92		2193	2249	2305	2364	2423	2484	2547	2611	2677	2745	2814	2885	2958	3033	3109	3188	3268							
93		2243	2299	2356	2415	2475	2537	2600	2665	2731	2799	2869	2941	3014	3089	3166	3245	3326	3409	3494					
94				2408	2467	2528	2590	2654	2719	2786	2855	2925	2997	3071	3147	3224	3304	3385	3468	3554					
95				2461	2521	2582	2645	2709	2775	2842	2912	2982	3055	3129	3205	3283	3363	3445	3528	3614					
96						2637	2701	2765	2832	2900	2969	3041	3114	3188	3265	3343	3423	3505	3590	3676	3764	3854			
97						2694	2757	2823	2890	2958	3028	3100	3173	3248	3325	3404	3485	3567	3652	3738	3827	3918			
98								2881	2949	3018	3088	3160	3234	3310	3387	3466	3547	3630	3715	3802	3891	3982	4075	4170	
99								2941	3009	3078	3149	3222	3296	3372	3450	3530	3611	3695	3780	3867	3956	4047	4141	4236	
100								3002	3071	3141	3212	3285	3360	3436	3514	3594	3676	3760	3845	3933	4022	4114	4207	4303	4401

N.B. All weights expressed in grams.

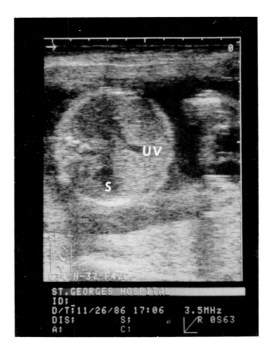

Figure 9.3   An ultrasound scan of a transverse section of a fetal abdomen at the correct level at which to measure the abdominal circumference (AC). The stomach (S) and a short segment of the umbilical vein (UV) are visible. The circumference is usually measured by means of on-screen calipers. This 24 week fetus had a weight estimate of 830 g. This was derived from Table 9.3 using a BPD = 67 mm and an AC = 197 mm

9.6.1.1   ABSOLUTE

1. Thyroid disease.
2. Cardiac disease.
3. Severe hypertension (more than 160/110 mmHg).
4. Sickle cell disease.
5. Chorio-amnionitis.
6. Patients taking monoamine oxidase inhibitors.

9.6.1.2   RELATIVE

1. Advanced labour (more than 4 cm cervical dilatation).
2. Antepartum haemorrhage. Tocolytic agents cause a maternal tachycardia so reduce the patient's ability to cope with blood loss.
3. Maternal diabetes mellitus (see Chapter 27).

9.6.2 Regimen for intravenous ritodrine

1. Warn the patient that the drug may cause her to feel anxious and that she may experience palpitations.
2. Dilute 50 mg ritodrine in 1 l of Hartmann's solution and administer it via an infusion pump through a 16 gauge cannula.
3. Start the infusion at 20 drops min^{-1} (50 µg min^{-1}) and double the rate every 15 min until:
    a. Uterine activity is suppressed. An effective rate is usually 150–300 µg min^{-1}
    b. The maternal pulse exceeds 140 beats min^{-1}.
    c. The systolic blood pressure exceeds 160 mmHg.
4. During the infusion the following observations should be recorded:
    a. Maternal pulse and blood pressure every 15 min.
    b. Fetal heart rate and uterine activity should be continuously recorded by external CTG.
5. Maintain a strict fluid balance chart.
6. Test all urine produced for glucose and ketones.
7. If the infusion is maintained for more than 24 h check the serum electrolytes.

9.7 STEROID THERAPY

Steroid therapy has been statistically shown to reduce the incidence of and the deaths from respiratory distress syndrome between the gestations of 28–32 weeks. From 32–34 weeks the value just fails to reach significance. It should be stressed that these results are based on statistical analysis and whilst helping the clinician to plan, the general strategy for the management of preterm labour treatment must be individualized.

9.7.1 Regimen

12 mg β-Methasone should be given by i.m. immediately the decision has been made that preterm delivery is likely. Repeat the dose 12 h later. In order to achieve maximum benefit delivery should be delayed for a further 24 h. Dexamethasone is often used instead of β-methasone at a dose of 4 mg, every 8 h for 48 h. It has no particular advantages over β-methasone and takes 24 h longer to administer. The course of steroids is valid for seven days and should be repeated if the patient is still felt to be at risk of preterm delivery.

9.7.2 Contraindications

1. Evidence of chorio-amnionitis.
2. Severe hypertension.
3. Maternal cardiac disease.
4. Asymmetrical intra-uterine growth retardation.

9.8   SUBSEQUENT MANAGEMENT

If:

1. Tocolysis is contraindicated or fails. As soon as the patient is in labour and the presenting part is engaged the membranes should be ruptured and a fetal scalp electrode should be attached. Appropriate analgesia should be advised (see Section 9.5).
2. Tocolysis is successful. Keep the patient on the labour ward with continuous monitoring whilst the ritodrine infusion is in progress. Having stopped uterine activity for 12 h the infusion rate can gradually be reduced until it is stopped. Some obstetricians like to replace the infusion with oral therapy which is commenced 2 h before stopping the infusion at a dose of 10 mg every 3 h both day and night.
3. Labour starts again within 48 h. A further attempt at tocolysis should be made using the same regimen in order to give the steroids chance to exert their maximum effect.
4. Labour starts again more than 48 h later. This is a difficult situation and two courses of action are possible:
   a. Attempt further tocolysis. Statistically the chances of usefully prolonging the pregnancy are small but on an individual patient basis it may be successful. Care must be taken, however, because prolonged use of ritodrine especially in combination with steroids may lead to maternal pulmonary oedema.
   b. Allow delivery with full monitoring.

9.9   DELIVERY

9.9.1   Breech presentation at less than 32 weeks gestation

All footling breech presentations should be delivered by Caesarean section. Many would advocate delivering all breech presentations at less than 32 weeks gestation by Caesarean section for the following reasons:

1. The preterm breech is a poor presenting part so cord prolapse at ARM/SRM is not uncommon.
2. The small breech trunk may slip through an incompletely dilated cervix with subsequent head entrapment.
3. The delay in delivery of the fetal head that occurs in all breech deliveries results in a high incidence of asphyxia which the preterm infant tolerates less well.
4. The amount of handling necessary for breech delivery results in excessive bruising.

The mode of delivery, however, remains controversial and for deliveries at less than 28 weeks gestation when the lower segment is barely formed a modified classical Caesarean section (De Lee incision) may be necessary if head entrapment and excessive handling is to be avoided.

9.9.2   Cephalic presentation at more than 25 weeks (600 g)

These patients will normally be allowed to deliver vaginally with full electronic monitoring and early recourse to Caesarean section for fetal distress.

9.9.3   Conduct of a normal delivery for a preterm infant

1.   The delivery should be conducted by a senior midwife (experienced staff nurse or sister) or by an obstetrician of registrar grade or above. The more preterm the infant the greater should be the experience of the person performing the delivery. If the delivery is being performed by a midwife the obstetric registrar/senior registrar should be present throughout the second stage.
2.   The neonatal paediatrician should be called well in advance of the delivery so that all the equipment can be checked.
3.   The aims of the delivery are to allow the fetal head to descend onto the perineum and then to have as short a period in the second stage as possible (about 30 min). It is during active pushing that the fetus becomes most acidotic. In order to achieve this short pushing second stage:
     a.   If the patient has an epidural do not allow it to wear off in the second stage. This allows fetal head descent in the absence of maternal effort. Pushing should commence when the presenting part is visible.
     b.   Perform an elective episiotomy. This reduces the time the fetus spends in the pushing second stage.
     c.   Do not perform an elective forceps delivery. There is no evidence that this benefits the fetus and forceps are not designed for preterm infants. Indications for forceps delivery are as for the term fetus (see Chapter 26).
     d.   The Ventouse is contraindicated in all preterm infants because of the substantial risk of cephalhaematoma formation.

9.9.4   Immediate postnatal management

If possible the parents should be allowed a brief cuddle before their baby is taken to NICU. The father should be encouraged to accompany the baby to the unit. As soon as her condition allows the mother should be taken to visit her baby. If she is not able to visit, a Polaroid photograph is usually very welcome and if the hospital has video facilities the mother may be able to watch her baby on a television monitor.

Chapter 10

Preterm, Premature Rupture of the Membranes

10.1   INTRODUCTION

Premature rupture of the membranes (PROM) refers to rupture of the membranes before the onset of labour. If this occurs at less than 37 weeks gestation if is referred to as preterm, premature rupture of the membranes (PPROM).

The decision to be made in cases of PPROM is whether there should be immediate delivery, possibly exposing the baby to the risks of prematurity or whether the patient should be managed conservatively with the possible risks of chorio-amnionitis. There is much controversy over management even within single hospitals so individual consultants' practices must be known. The following are guidelines to possible methods of management.

10.2   CONFIRMING THE DIAGNOSIS OF RUPTURED MEMBRANES

If the patient has a history suggestive of SRM *vaginal examination must be avoided* because of the risk of causing an ascending infection.

10.2.1 Method

1. Record the patient's temperature and pulse rate.
2. Palpate the abdomen to determine the fetal lie, position and size.
3. Perform a *sterile* speculum examination.
4. Confirmation of rupture of membranes is by one or all of the following means:
    a. Amniotic fluid is seen pouring out of the cervix either spontaneously or in response to a little fundal pressure. Amniotic fluid has a peculiar smell which is readily recognizable after a few days on the labour ward.
    b. pH testing. This is usually performed by means of a nitrazine stick test. Normal vaginal secretions have a pH of 4.5–5.5 and the stick remains yellow whereas amniotic fluid has a pH of 7.0–7.5 and turns the stick dark blue. Sperm, cervical secretions, infected urine and antiseptic creams may be alkaline and give a false positive reading.
    c. Microscopy. A direct wet preparation may reveal fetal hair, vernix or meconium whilst allowing amniotic fluid to dry on a glass slide produces ferning. This is a crystallized pattern seen under the microscope and is due to the high content of sodium chloride in amniotic fluid.
    d. Ultrasound. This may demonstrate oligohydramnios.
    e. A pad test. If the patient is not in labour and no amniotic fluid is observed she should be asked to walked around the labour ward wearing a sanitary towel. Inspection of the towel a few hours later may reveal the peculiar odour of amniotic fluid.
5. Take a swab from the cervix and collect as much amniotic fluid as possible via a sterile syringe and a sterile kwill (usually used for drawing up drugs). Send both to the laboratory for immediate microscopy and subsequent culture.

10.3 MANAGEMENT

10.3.1 PPROM after 34 weeks gestation

In these cases the risk of infection probably outweighs the risks of prematurity and the patient should be delivered once the diagnosis is confirmed. A vaginal examination may now be performed and a fetal scalp electrode should be attached. Labour should be induced with an intravenous syntocinon infusion (see Section 7.3.3). The following exceptions apply:

1. Patients admitted late at night. Having excluded a cord prolapse and infection (via direct microscopy) these patients may be allowed to sleep overnight and be induced early the next morning.
2. Patients with active genital herpes simplex virus infection. If the membranes have been ruptured for less than 4 h these patients should be delivered by Caesarean section because of the risk of the neonate acquiring the infection. After this time the risk of ascending infection are substantial and there is therefore no benefit of delivery by Caesarean section.

3. Those patients with β- haemolytic streptococci on direct microscopy. These patients should be induced immediately by means of a syntocinon infusion (see Section 7.3.3) and labour should be covered with 500 mg of ampicillin i.v. every 6 h. The paediatricians should be informed and the baby should be started on parenteral penicillin immediately after delivery.
4. Those patients who request no interference. The possible risk of infection should be explained to the mother and recorded in the notes. The mother's wishes should then be complied with and she should be managed conservatively as described below.

10.3.2 PPROM at less than 34 weeks gestation

Each case must be considered on its own merits but the following are possible lines of action:

1. *In utero* transfer to a hospital with a NICU. This should certainly be considered for all women of less than 30 weeks gestation unless delivery *en route* was likely.
2. Conservative treatment.
    a.   In order for this to be successful vaginal examinations must be avoided. Having confirmed the diagnosis by sterile speculum examination the patient is admitted to the antenatal ward and the following observations are performed:
        (i)   Four-hourly temperature and pulse.
        (ii) Twice daily CTG.
        (iii) Three times a week white cell count.
        (iv) Twice weekly low vaginal swabs.
        (v)   Weekly ultrasound examination to measure fetal growth and estimate the amount of amniotic fluid remaining.
    b. The woman should be encouraged to be in bed as much as possible but should be allowed up to the toilet and to bath.
    c. Delivery is indicated for:
        (i)   Evidence of chorio-amnionitis. This is suggested by a rise in maternal pulse and/or temperature, fetal tachycardia, a tender uterus with a foul smelling discharge or a rise in maternal white cell count.
        (ii) Maturity. This will depend upon local views but delivery at or after 34 weeks is usually justified.
        (iii) The spontaneous onset of labour. Although each case should be discussed on its own merits it is usually unwise to attempt tocolysis in patients who have been managed conservatively and then go into labour.
    d. Contraindications to conservative management:
        (i)   Evidence of chorio-amnionitis.
        (ii) Evidence of genital herpes.
        (iii) Evidence of β- haemolytic streptococci infection. Although not all would agree it is probably wise to deliver such patients immediately under ampicillin cover (see Section 10.3.1).
3. Amniocentesis. It is now widely believed that many cases of PPROM are due to infection of the membranes. If infection is not present at the time of PPROM ascending infection probably does not occur unless a vaginal examination has been performed. As the clinical evidence of chorio-amnionitis occurs late in the course of the disease amniocentesis is used to detect infection.

10.3.2.1   MANAGEMENT

1. Having confirmed the diagnosis of PPROM by sterile speculum examination rest the patient in bed for 4 h with her feet elevated to allow the amniotic fluid to accumulate.
2. Perform an amniocentesis under ultrasound guidance aiming for the largest accessible pool of amniotic fluid. This should be performed by an operator who is skilled at amniocentesis and the success rate for obtaining fluid should be more than 90 per cent.
3. Send the fluid for direct microscopy and for estimation of the lecithin–sphingomyelin (L/S) ratio and for the presence of phosphatydylglycerol (PTG) if possible. Management depends on the results as follows:
   a. Organisms seen on microscopy—delivery.
   b. L/S ratio >2 (and preferably PTG present)—delivery.
   c. Neither of the above—conservative management as detailed above.

10.4   MANAGEMENT OF CHORIO-AMNIONITIS

This is usually diagnosed by one or more of the following:

1. A maternal temperature and tachycardia with no other obvious cause.
2. A tender uterus and/or a foul smelling discharge.
3. A fetal tachycardia.
4. A rise in maternal white cell count.
5. The presence of organisms on microscopy of the amniotic fluid, obtained by amniocentesis.

10.4.1   Management

1. Obtain a high vaginal, cervical and throat swab, MSSU and a blood culture.
2. Expedite delivery preferably by stimulating labour with a syntocinon infusion. It is preferable to avoid Caesarean section under these circumstances because of the high incidence of subsequent pelvic sepsis and possible tubal damage. Caesarean section, however, is indicated for:
   a. Fetal distress.
   b. Preterm breech or other abnormal lie.
   c. Failed induction.
3. Do not give antibiotics until after delivery unless the infection is thought to be due to β-haemolytic streptococci. A delay of 12 h in starting antibiotics will not do the mother any harm but it denies the paediatricians the opportunity to obtain positive cultures from the baby. After delivery give iv broad spectrum antibiotics (such as 500 mg ampicillin or 500 mg cephradine) together with 500 mg metronidazole iv to the mother. If the patient is delivered by Caesarean section these should be commenced immediately after the cord is clamped and in all cases intravenous therapy should be continued for 48 h before starting oral therapy for a further five days.

Chapter 11
Pre-eclampsia and Eclampsia

11.1 INTRODUCTION

Pre-eclampsia is a condition peculiar to pregnancy characterized by hypertension and proteinuria, which may lead to *eclampsia* or epileptiform convulsions. The terminology and classification of hypertensive disorders in pregnancy is confusing and universal agreement regarding definitions has not yet been reached.

The condition is of unknown aetiology but probably has an immunological basis. It is almost exclusively found in women in their first pregnancy, and is particularly common at each end of the maternal age range. It may present for the first time as an antepartum, intrapartum or postpartum event, and usually resolves rapidly after the pregnancy has ended.

The term *fulminating pre-eclampsia* is used for the situation of a rapid rise of blood pressure accompanied by symptoms of impending eclampsia. These symptoms are:

1. Headache. Dragging headache, worse on standing.
2. Epigastric pain due to stretching of the liver capsule.
3. Visual defects (scotomata). These are due to oedema of the optic nerve, and are missing parts of the visual fields. Floaters, blurred edges or coloured rims to objects are not the result of impending eclampsia.

11.2 PRINCIPLES OF MANAGEMENT

1. Close observation and monitoring of the fetal and maternal condition.
2. Awareness of possible complications and therefore early recognition and treatment of abnormal clinical signs.
3. Delivery of the fetus at an appropriate time, and by the appropriate route.

11.3 COMPLICATIONS OF PRE-ECLAMPSIA

1. Maternal.
    a. Cerebrovascular accidents.
    b. Renal impairment leading to oliguria and renal failure.
    c. Hepatic damage, which may result in rupture of the capsule in severe cases.
    d. DIC (see Chapter 14).
    e. Eclampsia.
    f. Placental abruption.
2. Fetal.
    a. Intra-uterine growth retardation.
    b. Fetal distress in labour.
    c. Preterm delivery as a result of obstetric intervention.
    d. Fetal death due to placental abruption, or asphyxia in labour.

11.4 ASSESSMENT OF THE PATIENT

11.4.1 History

Specific enquiry should be made concerning the symptoms shown in Table 11.1.

Table 11.1   Symptoms for specific enquiry

Symptom	Possible pathology
Nausea and vomiting	
Headache	Cerebral oedema
Visual disturbances	
Epigastric pain	Stretching of liver capsule
Vaginal bleeding	Placental abruption
Abdominal pain	Placental abruption or spontaneous labour
Reduced fetal movements	Fetal compromise

11.4.2   Examination

Specific signs and their pathologies are shown in Table 11.2.

Table 11.2   Signs for specific examination

Specific signs	Possible pathology
i. *Oedema* Facial and finger	Worsening pre-eclampsia
ii. *Neurological status* Hyper-reflexia Clonus	Cerebral oedema plus impending eclampsia
iii. *Cardiovascular system* Elevated arterial blood pressure	Worsening pre-eclampsia plus impending eclampsia
iv. *Abdomen* Epigastric tenderness	Stretching of the liver capsule
Uterine tenderness	Placental abruption
Low fundal height and clinically small fetus	IUGR
Fetal heart rate abnormalities	Fetal distress

11.4.3   Investigations

1.   An intravenous cannula should be inserted, and blood taken for:
    a.   Haemoglobin and platelet count.
    b.   Clotting screen (at least platelets, thrombin and prothrombin time).
    c.   Group and save serum.
    d.   Urea and electrolytes.

2. MSU
3. 24 h Urine collection for total protein estimation.
4. Abdominal ultrasound, to assess fetal growth and obtain an estimate of fetal weight and amniotic fluid volume.

11.5 NURSING CARE AND OBSERVATIONS

The patient should be cared for by a single trained midwife who never leaves the delivery room. She should be nursed in a quiet room, but darkness should be avoided as it is important to be able to see the patient's colour, level of consciousness, and adequacy of respiratory movement. Severe headache, nausea and vomiting and visual disturbances signify cerebral irritation and impending eclampsia. In the case of patients with severe pre-eclampsia or those who have already suffered an epileptic fit, a mouth gag (see Figure 11.1) and an ampoule of 20 mg diazepam already drawn up into a syringe and labelled appropriately should be kept available in the room.

The fetal heart should be monitored by continuous cardiotocography.

Maternal blood pressure and pulse rate should be recorded every 15 min. If the pre-eclampsia is severe (i.e. diastolic blood pressure >110 mmHg), an in-dwelling urethral catheter should be inserted so that hourly urine output can be recorded. The severe

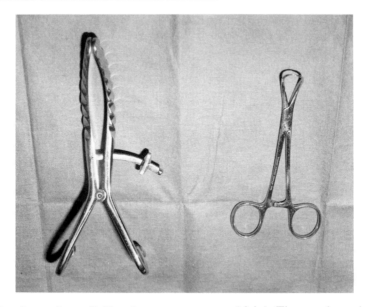

Figure 11.1   A mouth gag (left) and a tongue extractor (right). The mouth gag is placed between the patient's molar teeth and as the handles are squeezed together the patient's mouth will open. If necessary the tongue can be prevented from falling back into the throat by means of the tongue extractor, the tooth of which is put through the patient's tongue

pre-eclamptic is likely to require insertion of a central venous pressure line to enable fluid balance to be accurately monitored particularly if urine output deteriorates (see below). Tendon reflexes should be tested every hour.

11.6 SPECIFIC THERAPY

11.6.1 Antihypertensive therapy

These drugs are specifically indicated in fulminating pre-eclampsia when maternal blood pressure is persistently equal to or in excess of 160/110 mmHg (i.e. on two readings at least 30 min apart). Simply lowering the blood pressure will not remove the risk of eclampsia, and therefore the patient who exhibits neurological signs (see above) should also be given anticonvulsant therapy. The aim of hypotensive therapy is to achieve a diastolic blood pressure of not less than 90 mmHg. If further hypotension occurs placental perfusion will be jeopardized, and fetal distress or death may result.

11.6.1.1 HYDRALAZINE

Hydralazine causes a fall in systolic and diastolic pressure. It acts directly on the smooth muscle of arteriolar walls to cause vasodilatation. In theory, therefore, it should not cause decreased placental perfusion. It should be given by intravenous injection as absorption from muscle is delayed and erratic in pre-eclampsia.

Side-effects include tachycardia, flushing, nasal irritation, tremor, headaches, nausea and vomiting. These signs may mimic those of cerebral irritation, confusing the clinical picture.

Dose

We recommend initial treatment with a bolus of 10 mg hydralazine iv given slowly, with blood pressure recording every 5 min thereafter. This is less likely to result in overdosage and unpleasant side effects than the continuous infusion regimen formerly advocated. Boluses can be repeated every 20 min as necessary.

11.6.1.2 DIAZOXIDE

This drug acts by a similar mechanism to hydralazine. Its drawbacks include a very rapid hypotensive effect, salt and water retention and hyperuricaemia, and suppression of uterine activity. It may also cause respiratory depression in the neonate when given to the mother in conjunction with chlormethiazole. It has been less extensively used than hydralazine but may be necessary where this has failed to lower the blood pressure.

The recommended dose is 30 mg iv every minute until the desired hypotensive effect is achieved, monitoring the blood pressure continuously.

11.6.2 Anticonvulsant therapy

Specific anticonvulsant therapy is indicated in fulminating pre-eclampsia when signs of cerebral oedema or hyper-reflexia and/or clonus are demonstrable. There are unavoidable drawbacks of anticonvulsants in that they have side effects on the baby (see below).

11.6.2.1 DIAZEPAM

This benzodiazepine acts rapidly by a direct central depressant mechanism. It is rapidly transferred across the placenta and causes loss of baseline variability of the fetal heart trace (see Figure 15.2). The neonate may exhibit hypoglycaemia, hypotonia and hypothermia, all of which should be anticipated and therefore dealt with appropriately. There are no long-term detrimental effects on the neonate.

An initial dose of 10–20 mg is given intravenously, followed by an infusion at a rate of 10 mg h^{-1}. Evidence has suggested that this is the dose necessary to prevent eclamptic fits.

Despite its neonatal side effects diazepam is effective at preventing and treating fits which carry a 30 per cent risk of fetal death.

11.6.2.2 CHLORMETHIAZOLE

This drug also acts rapidly. It is given as a 0.8 per cent solution intravenously at a rate of 4–8 ml min^{-1} until drowsiness occurs. Superficial thrombophlebitis often occurs at the site of the iv cannula. The therapeutic margin between adequate sedation and loss of consciousness is narrow, so particular attention to level of consciousness and respiratory effort should be made. It is a sedative rather than an anticonvulsant. It crosses the placenta and causes neonatal respiratory depression.

11.6.2.3 MAGNESIUM SULPHATE

This drug is not used extensively in the UK. It acts by depressing neuromuscular transmission and has no sedative or hypotensive effect.

10 g magnesium sulphate is added to 1 ℓ Hartmann's solution and 4 g (400 ml) is given iv over 10 min followed by 1–2 g hourly (100–200 ml) iv. Serum magnesium levels must be checked every 4 h, to maintain a therapeutic level of 3–4 mmol ℓ^{-1} (6–8 meq ℓ^{-1}). If urinary output is less than 30 ml h^{-1}, levels should be checked more frequently, and 5 mmol ℓ^{-1} (10 meq ℓ^{-1}) should not be exceeded. It is excreted by the kidney, and therefore renal impairment will affect its metabolism. It potentiates succinyl choline and curare and therefore if general anaesthesia is later required, the anaesthetist should be aware that this drug has been used. It often decreases or stops uterine activity.

Magnesium sulphate may have a marked depressive effect on maternal respiration but this is unlikely to occur if the knee jerks are present. The antidote is 1 g calcium gluconate intravenously.

11.7 MANAGEMENT OF ECLAMPSIA

Eclampsia is more common in the unbooked patient, but in only about one-quarter of patients will it have been preceded by pre-eclampsia. The maternal risks from eclampsia are proportional to the number of fits, so prompt treatment and control is essential.

In the event of an eclamptic fit, senior obstetric and anaesthetic staff should be summoned as quickly as possible, meanwhile:

1. The patient should be turned on her side and the airway should be cleared by opening the jaw with a mouth gag, pulling the tongue forward and aspirating any vomitus (see Figure 11.1). An oropharyngeal airway is then inserted.
2. A dose of 10 mg diazepam is given slowly i.v. and repeated after 10 min if convulsions continue. The patient is observed carefully for her level of consciousness and respiratory effort.
3. If the patient becomes cyanosed, oxygen at 4.5 ℓ min^{-1} is administered via a face mask.
4. If cardiac arrest occurs, cardio-respiratory resuscitation should be commenced immediately.
5. Hypotensive and anticonvulsant maintenance therapy should be instituted as described above.
6. Delivery should take place as soon as the patient's condition has stabilized (see below), because the occurrence of eclampsia signifies the end-stage of the condition, and the maternal and fetal risk does not justify further prolonging the pregnancy.

Immediate Caesarean section is the usual course of action, but selected patients may have labour induced if the following conditions apply:

a. The cervix is very favourable (Bishops score >6, see p. 66).
b. The maternal condition is stable.
c. There is no fetal distress.
d. There is a cephalic presentation.
e. No further fits occur.

11.8 LABOUR AND DELIVERY

11.8.1 Timing and mode of delivery

All patients with eclampsia and severe pre-eclampsia warranting intravenous agents should be delivered. The only exception to this is if blood pressure can be sufficiently controlled in a severe pre-eclamptic such that *in utero* transfer to a regional centre with a neonatal intensive care unit may be considered. The decision as to whether it is safe for the patient to be moved, however, must be made at the most senior level.

The aim to attempt vaginal delivery as Caesarean section complicates the clinical situation and delays recovery from the pathological process. Caesarean section is positively indicated for the following reasons:

1. Failed induction of labour or labour that is unlikely to result in delivery within 6–8 h.
2. The preterm breech or other fetal malpresentation.
3. Fetal distress.
4. Placental abruption.
5. Difficulty in control of maternal blood pressure.

11.8.2   Use of epidural analgesia

Epidural analgesia in severe pre-eclampsia and eclampsia is associated with certain hazards but may effectively be used if precautions are taken. The hazards include:

1. The possibility of a clotting disorder. This must always be excluded in pre-eclampsia or eclampsia before an epidural block is sited.
2. The possibility of sudden severe hypotension due to peripheral vasodilatation. This may jeopardize placental perfusion and lead to acute fetal distress. This effect can be prevented by preloading with 500 ml of Hartmann's solution and reducing the dose of hypotensive agents.

11.8.3   Augmentation of contractions

If the decision is made to induce labour it is sensible to start syntocinon as soon as the membranes are ruptured. Accurate fluid balance must obviously be kept and continuous fetal monitoring is mandatory.

   Nursing care and observations should be continued as described above.

11.8.4   The second stage

Pushing in the second stage should not be permitted as this causes a marked a rise in maternal blood pressure. An elective forceps delivery at full dilatation and after a short second stage is therefore the rule.

11.8.5   The third stage

Syntometrine should be avoided in the third stage as it results in further elevation of the blood pressure. Five to ten units of intravenous syntocinon as a bolus should be used as an alternative.

11.9   THE PUERPERIUM

A significant risk of eclampsia in the pre-eclamptic patient persists for the first 48 h after delivery. Up to a third of patients who have eclamptic fits will have their first fit in the puerperium. In addition the maternal risks resulting from the hypertension persist. Close monitoring of the maternal condition over this period of time should therefore be maintained.

11.9.1   Observations

1. Blood pressure and pulse. These should be recorded every quarter of an hour and the blood pressure should be maintained at levels between 140/90 mmHg and 160/110 mmHg. As the baby is now delivered almost any intravenous agent may be used, most commonly hydralazine. If control is not achieved with hydralazine an infusion of labetalol is a good choice as the drug may be given orally when

appropriate. The solution is made up by diluting 40 ml (200 mg of labetalol) in 160 ml of 5 per cent dextrose using a paediatric burette. This gives a concentration of 1 mg of labetalol per ml and should be infused at an initial rate of 20 ml h^{-1} (20 mg h^{-1}). The dose may be doubled every 30 min up to a maximum concentration of 160 ml h^{-1} (160 mg h^{-1}).

2. Respiratory rate. This should be recorded every 15 min and should be above 10 per min. If the rate is lower than this it may be necessary to reduce the infusion of diazepam or to initiate endotracheal intubation and intermittent positive pressure ventilation.

3. Level of consciousness. This is a guide to the dose of anticonvulsant needed. It is most important that the patient is sufficiently conscious to maintain her gag reflex in order to prevent inhalation of any vomitus.

4. The patients reflexes should be tested hourly. Hyper-reflexia and clonus suggest impending eclampsia and an intravenous infusion of diazepam should be started or if already in progress the infusion rate should be increased.

5. Urinary output. This should be measured hourly and should be maintained at more than 20 ml h^{-1}. The management of oliguria is detailed in Section 11.10.

The patient should be nursed in the left lateral position and should have a constant attendant.

Recovery from the pathological process is usually indicated by a diuresis. This occurs 6–12 h after vaginal delivery, but may be delayed for 24–36 h if Caesarean section has been necessary. The reason for this delay is that the metabolic response to surgery results in an increase in the production of antidiuretic hormone (ADH).

If fits occur after the first 24 h of the puerperium another possible cause should be sought. Sleepiness, headache, vomiting and a hemiparesis should be sought as these indicate a cerebrovascular accident.

As a general rule anticonvulsant therapy can usually be reduced after the first 12 h and stopped completely by 24 h. Patients commonly remain hypertensive but may be given oral medication after the first 48 h. It is not uncommon for them to continue to need therapy until discharge from hospital. If they are discharged on oral therapy they should be reviewed fortnightly by their general practitioner and the dose reduced or stopped as appropriate. The use of the combined oral contraceptive is not contraindicated following delivery as long as the blood pressure has returned to normal.

11.10 MANAGEMENT OF OLIGURIA

This is defined as an hourly urine production rate of less than 20 ml h^{-1} (500 ml day^{-1}). This is the minimal amount of urine necessary to excrete the products of metabolism. After delivery if the patient produces less than 20 ml of urine for 2 h the following steps should be taken:

1. Check that the Foley catheter is not blocked either by observing urine dribbling down the tubing or by flushing the catheter with a bladder syringe.

2. An anaesthetist or appropriately experienced person should insert a central venous pressure line. Once the line is inserted a portable chest X-ray should be taken to

ensure that the tip of the line has entered the right atrium. An additional check on this is that the meniscus in the vertical column should move as the patient breathes. The method of using these central venous pressure line is detailed in Figure 11.2. The normal central venous pressure measured at the sternal angle (angle of Louis) in pregnancy is +4 to +10 cm of water. Most pre-eclamptics and eclamptics are relatively volume-depleted and are therefore in pre-renal failure.

3. Send blood for urea and electrolyte measurement and test the urine for specific gravity. Tests of plasma and urine osmolality and electrolytes are not widely available but may be helpful and their interpretation is detailed in Table 11.3.

4. Measure the central venous pressure and if it is less than +4 cm of water give 1 ℓ

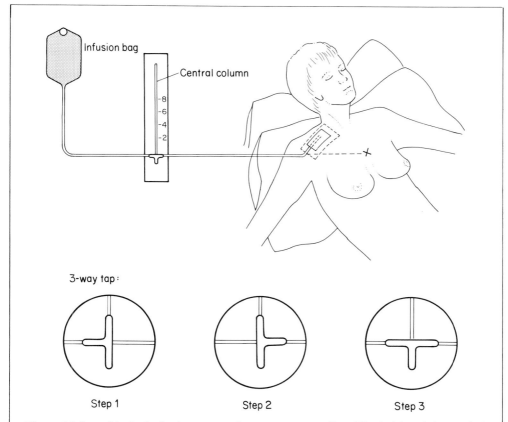

Figure 11.2   Method of using a central venous pressure line. The height of the vertical tube is adjusted until the bubble in the attached spirit level indicates that it is horizontal to the sterno-manubrial angle (angle of Louis). The central venous pressure (CVP) is measured as follows. Step 1: Fill the central column of fluid from the infusion bag. Step 2: Alter the three way tap so that the connection is now between the central column of fluid and the patient. Allow the fluid in the central column to fall until it is stable. Record the lowest level as the CVP. Step 3: Move the three way tap until the infusion bag is connected directly to the patient

Table 11.3   Interpretation of tests commonly used in patients with oliguria

	Pre-renal failure	Acute tubular necrosis
Urine specific gravity	>1.010	1.010
Urinary osmolality (MOSM kg^{-1} H$_2$O)	> 300	< 300
Urine sodium concentration (mmol ℓ^{-1})	< 20	> 20
U/P creatinine	> 40	< 40
U/P urea	> 10	< 2
U/P osmolality	>1.5	<1.1

U/P = urine/plasma

of Hartmann's solution over 30 min. If the CVP is still not more than 4 cm of water give 500 ml of Haemaccel.

5. Following elevation of the central venous pressure the patient should respond by increasing urine output over the next hour to more than 20 ml h^{-1}.

    If this does not happen then the patient either has acute tubular necrosis (ATN) or renal failure as a result of the pre-eclamptic process. ATN is reversible in its early stages by correcting circulating plasma volume as described above and by the administration of diuretics. Therefore give 40 mg of frusemide intravenously slowly. This should result in a diuresis of over 30 ml h^{-1} within the next hour. If this fails to occur give 200 mg of frusemide every 20 min to a maximum of 2 g. If diuresis does not occur following this the patient is in renal failure and the help of a nephrologist should be sought.

    Do not give mannitol. Although many people use mannitol in early acute ATN if the patient is in renal failure they are unable to excrete it and therefore cardiac failure may occur.

6. Principles of management of renal failure.
    a.   Give the patient their hourly urine output plus 20 ml of 5 per cent glucose intravenously each hour.
    b.   Check urea, electrolytes and creatinine daily.
    c.   Weigh the patient daily.
    d.   Give the patient a high protein diet.

If the renal failure is due to ATN two to three days following the acute insult a diuretic phase will occur and this signals recovery. It is important that during the diuretic phase fluid replacement keeps pace with the urinary loss.

    If the patient is in renal failure from other causes (rare) they should be managed with the help of a nephrologist.

11.11 MANAGEMENT OF PULMONARY OEDEMA

Pulmonary oedema in the hypertensive patient can occur by several mechanisms:

1. Increased intravascular hydrostatic pressure.
2. Increased capillary permeability.
3. Low vascular oncotic pressure due to low plasma albumin.

If pulmonary oedema occurs it does so 5–24 h following delivery and is particularly likely to occur following the administration of significant volumes of intravenous fluid.

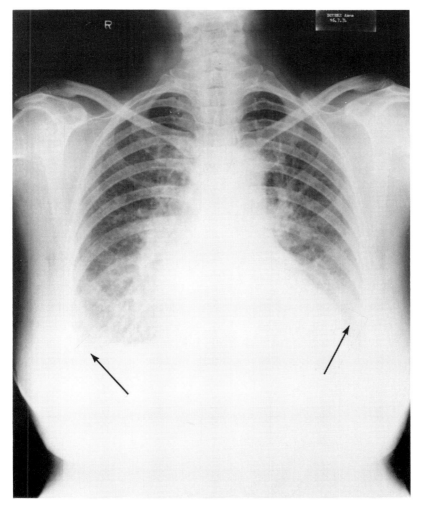

Figure 11.3   A chest X-ray demonstrating pulmonary oedema. The vascular markings are prominent and the costal angles are blunted due to small pleural effusions (arrows)

11.11.1 Diagnosis

This is based on the following features:

1. Clinical respiratory distress.
2. Hypoxaemia (pO_2 less than 70 mmHg).
3. Confirmatory X-ray evidence which includes increased vasular markings, Curley B-lines, pleural effusions causes blunting of the subcostal angle (see Figure 11.3).

11.11.2 Management

1. Sit the patient upright and administer oxygen via a face mask at 4 ℓ min^{-1}.
2. Give 40 mg of frusemide intravenously.
3. Infuse 200 ml of 4.5 per cent salt-free albumin over a 30 min period.

In most patients this is all that is necessary. Failure to resond to this regime indicates that the patient should have her pulmonary artery wedge pressure (PAWP) measured.

11.11.3 Indications for PAWP

CVP measurement is a poor indicator of left ventricular preload particularly in severe pre-eclampsia. Measurement of PAWP is therefore indicated in the following circumstances:

1. When the above measures fail to produce a rapid improvement in the pulmonary function.
2. When colloid fluid has been administered to the severely pre-eclamptic patient prior to delivery. This may result in excessive movement of fluid from the extravascular space into the intravascular space immediately after delivery. This will raise hydrostatic pressure and combined with the low intravascular oncotic pressure may result in pulmonary oedema.
3. Persistent oliguria. The Swan–Ganz catheter for measurement of PAWP should be inserted by a skilled anaesthetist. Interpretation of the results also requires collaboration with an anaesthetist or an intensive care physician. In essence if the cause of the pulmonary oedema is myocardial failure there will be a raised PAWP.

Chapter 12
Antepartum Haemorrhage

12.1 INTRODUCTION

Antepartum haemorrhage (APH) is defined as bleeding from the genital tract after 28 weeks gestation. It occurs in about 3 per cent of all pregnancies. Its causes are as follows:

1. Placental abruption.
2. Placenta praevia.
3. Other placental causes and local causes.

The definition has not kept pace with the times and the management described below is applicable to all women thought to be carrying a potentially viable fetus (usually of more than 24 weeks gestation).

The management of APH does not initially follow the classical lines of history, examination and investigations because the management of a major abruption is urgent.

12.2 MANAGEMENT OF ANTEPARTUM HAEMORRHAGE

Any woman admitted to the labour ward with a history of vaginal bleeding should have an *immediate* abdominal palpation. If the uterus is *woody hard* the fetal heart should be immediately sought with a Pinard's stethoscope or a Sonicaid fetal heart detector. If it is present the patient should be moved immediately to theatre and the obstetric registrar and anaesthetist should be called. The diagnosis is of a major abruption and prompt action is needed if the fetus is to be rescued.

12.2.1 Management of a major abruption with a live fetus

1. Call the obstetric registrar, the anaesthetist and the paediatrician. Order the theatre to be prepared.
2. Insert two large bore cannulae (at least 16 gauge) and start infusions of normal saline or Hartmann's solution.
3. Take blood for the following:
   a. Haemoglobin estimation
   b. Group and cross-match two units of blood
   c. Urea and electrolytes
   d. Clotting studies, to include:
      (i) Platelet count.
      (ii) FDPs.
      (iii) Thrombin time.
      (iv) Prothrombin time.
      (v) Fibrinogen titre (if available).
4. Send a request with the porter who takes the blood samples to the laboratory for two units of fresh frozen plasma (FFP).
5. On arrival in the operating theatre perform an immediate vaginal examination. If the cervix is fully dilated and the fetal head is judged to be sufficiently low in the pelvis perform a forceps delivery. If not, perform an immediate Caesarean section.
6. If excessive bleeding is encountered after delivery and the blood on the floor is not obviously clotting defrost two units of FFP and give it to the patient together with sufficient crystalloid to replace the lost volume.
7. At the conclusion of the operation ask the anaesthetist to insert a central venous pressure line whilst the patient is still under the general anaesthetic.
8. Insert a 12–14 FG Foley's catheter with a 5–10 ml balloon.
9. Start an infusion of 20 units of syntocinon in 500 ml of Hartmann's solution at 80 drops min^{-1}. Run this over the next 2 h in order to avoid a PPH.
10. Make the following observations following delivery:
   a. Maternal pulse—every 15 min.
   b. Blood pressure and CVP reading every 30 min. The position of the CVP line should be confirmed with a portable chest X-ray.
   c. Hourly urine output.
   d. The blood loss.

Further management of abnormal clotting is detailed in Chapter 14.

A urine output of less than 20 ml h^{-1} should be treated by volume replacement, either by crystalloids or Haemaccel until the CVP is between +4 cm and +8 cm water (above the sternal angle). If this does not result in an adequate diuresis in the next hour then give 40 mg frusemide. This should produce an increased urine output in the next hour, if not proceed as detailed for oliguria following pre-eclampsia (see

Section 11.10). Do *not* give mannitol in this situation as occasionally the abruption will cause acute cortical necrosis. The patient will be unable to excrete the drug and pulmonary oedema will result.

12.2.2 Management of a major abruption with a dead fetus

If the fetus is dead on admission or dies on the way to theatre proceed as above but do not perform a Caesarean section if the cervix is not fully dilated.

Labour usually progresses rapidly and delivery can be expected within 4–6 h. Vaginal examinations should be performed at two hourly intervals and if progress is not rapid a syntocinon infusion (see Section 7.3.3) should be commenced.

Make the same observations as detailed above during labour and if urine output falls below 20 ml h^{-1} insert a CVP line and measure the central venous pressure. Management is as detailed above.

After delivery start an infusion of syntocinon to prevent a PPH (as above).

12.3 MANAGEMENT OF ANTEPARTUM HAEMORRHAGE NOT DUE TO MAJOR ABRUPTION

If on admission the patient does not have a woody hard uterus and is not clinically shocked management should proceed along standard lines with the following points being noted.

12.3.1 History

1. Determine the gestational age and review the pregnancy to date.
2. Ask the patient to estimate the amount of blood loss and its colour. Red blood is fresh whereas brown blood is denatured and suggests that the bleeding is not recent.
3. Determine if the bleeding started after intercourse. Such bleeding usually suggests a local cause but may also be due to placenta praevia.
4. Find out if there was associated abdominal pain and if so its temporal relationship to the bleeding. Pain followed by a little brown bleeding suggests a small abruption whereas fresh red bleeding followed by pain suggests placenta praevia with associated uterine contractions.

12.3.2 Examination

1. Determine if the patient is shocked from her colour, blood pressure and pulse rate (see Chapter 16).
2. Palpate the abdomen particularly to determine:
   a. The presence of any uterine tenderness suggestive of a small abruption. This sign is not always elicited after an abruption when the placenta is posterior.
   b. The presence of uterine contractions.
   c. The size, lie and presentation of the fetus. A high presenting part may suggest a placenta praevia.

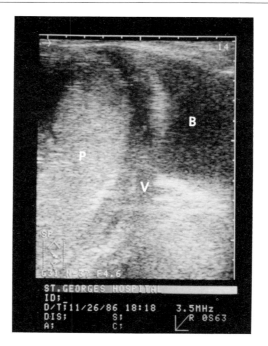

Figure 12.1 A longitudinal ultrasound scan demonstrating a major degree (type III) placenta praevia. (P = placenta, B = maternal bladder, V = vagina)

3. If possible perform a real time ultrasound examination on the labour ward to localize the placenta. If there is a placenta praevia (Figure 12.1) the bleeding is assumed to arise from this source. If the placenta is in the upper segment a speculum examination should be performed whilst the patient is still bleeding to determine whether the blood is coming through the cervical os (suggesting a placental cause) or whether there is a local lesion.

4. If a real time ultrasound machine is not immediately available a speculum examination may still be performed as the risk of provoking further bleeding from a placenta praevia is largely theoretical and it is important for future management to determine the source of the bleeding. However, a digital vaginal examination is contraindicated.

12.3.3 Investigations

Blood should be sent for:

1. Haemoglobin estimation.
2. Group and save serum (cross-match 2 units if the diagnosis is placenta praevia or the maternal pulse rate is more than 100 beats min^{-1}).
3. Rhesus group. Kleihauer test if the patient is rhesus negative.

12.3.4 Management

This depends upon the degree of the blood loss and the cause of the bleeding.

12.3.4.1 BLEEDING FROM PLACENTA PRAEVIA

1. Start an infusion of normal saline or Hartmann's via a large bore cannula (at least 16 gauge).
2. Cross-match two units of blood.
3. Monitor the fetus by means of external CTG.
4. Record maternal pulse and blood pressure, quarter hourly.

Outcome

Most patients will stop bleeding spontaneously. They should be given 500 i.u. of Anti-D if they are rhesus negative and transferred to an antenatal ward. Bedrest is usually advised for 24 h after the fresh bleeding has stopped. Two units of blood should be permanently cross-matched for that patient and kept in the labour ward blood refrigerator.

If the loss is estimated to exceed 500 ml the patient should be transfused and four more units of blood cross-matched. Delivery by Caesarean section is indicated for:

1. Excessive blood loss.
2. Fetal distress (rare).
3. The onset of spontaneous labour.

Placenta praevia is usually classified as illustrated in Figure 12.2. Types II (posterior), III and IV require delivery by Caesarean section.

12.3.4.2 BLEEDING FROM A LOCAL CAUSE

This is diagnosed at the time of speculum examination and may be due to:

1. Vaginal or cervical infections. The most common organisms are *Candida albicans* and *Trichomonas vaginalis*. The former is readily recognizable by characteristic cheesy white plaques on the vaginal walls which result in capillary bleeding when they are disturbed. The latter produces a frothy offensive green discharge. After taking a high vaginal swab they may be treated with clotrimazole pessaries (200 mg for three nights) or metronidazole 800 mg orally for three nights, respectively.
2. Cervical erosion (ectropion). This finding requires no treatment in pregnancy as it rarely produces severe bleeding but a cervical smear should be taken.
3. Cervical neoplasms. Small cervical polyps are best left alone since avulsion in pregnancy may cause substantial bleeding. Rarely, the source of bleeding will be overt carcinoma of the cervix. Although the blood loss from a carcinoma may be substantial it usually stops with bedrest and fluid replacement and emergency surgery or radiotherapy are almost never required.
4. Vaginal tears. These usually result from vigorous intercourse or masturbation with a foreign object. Epidural or general anaesthesia is usually required for repair.

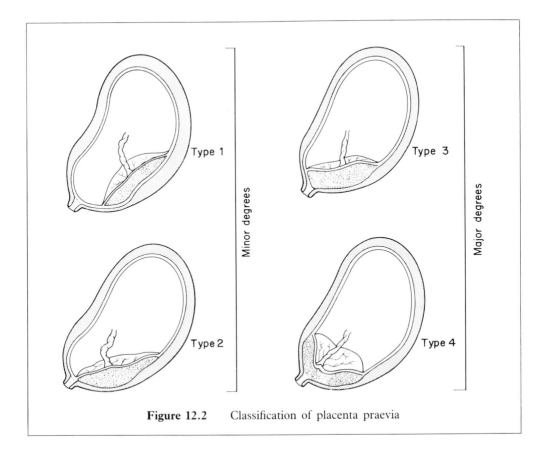

Figure 12.2   Classification of placenta praevia

12.3.4.3   BLEEDING OF UNDEFINED ORIGIN

The possible differential diagnoses include:

1. A small placental abruption.
2. Placenta circumvallate
3. Bleeding from a marginal sinus of the placenta.
4. Bleeding from vasa praevia. Bleeding from vasa praevia is rare but prompt recognition and delivery by Caesarean section may save the fetus. Diagnosis may be made from:
    a. A sinusoidal fetal heart rate trace (see Figure 15.4).
    b. Recognition that the blood is fetal in origin. This may be done by sending the blood for a Kleihauer test or more conveniently on the labour ward by use of sodium metasilicate tablets (Miles Laboratories, Stoke Poges, Bucks). These tablets are alkaline and will denature maternal but not fetal haemoglobin. They are crushed onto a glass slide and mixed with a drop of blood. If they stay red-pink the blood is fetal in origin; it they go dark brown it is maternal.

Management of the remaining conditions is conservative by means of bedrest until 24 h after the fresh bleeding has ceased and by assessment of fetal well-being by means of ultrasound and CTGs.

Note: All Rhesus negative patients that experience an APH should be given 500 i.u. Anti-D within 72 h of the bleeding. Blood should be sent for Kleihauer and further Anti-D may be advised by the blood bank if there has been a substantial feto–maternal haemorrhage.

Chapter 13

Postpartum Haemorrhage

13.1   DEFINITION

Postpartum haemorrhage (PPH) is defined as bleeding from the genital tract in excess of 500 ml after the delivery of the baby. If it occurs during the first 24 h, it is a primary PPH; if it occurs after this time it is a secondary PPH.

13.2   RISK FACTORS ASSOCIATED WITH PPH

1. Over-distension of the uterus.
    a.   Twin pregnancy.
    b.   Polyhydramnios.
    c.   Macrosomia.
2. Impaired myometrial contractility.
    a.   Multiparity. This is because myometrial fibres are successively replaced by fibrous tissue with increasing parity.
    b.   Placental abruption and placenta praevia. In the case of placental abruption blood clot in the myometrium will interfere with contractility. There may also be a coagulopathy.
    c.   Uterine fibroids
3. When there is a bleeding tendency.
    a.   Secondary to pre-eclampsia (Chapter 11).
        (i)   Intra-uterine death (Chapter 35).
        (ii) Placental abruption (Chapter 12).

(iii) Amniotic fluid embolism (Chapter 16).
   b. Von Willebrand's disease.
4. Past History of a PPH

In these groups of high-risk women, prophylaxis against a PPH should be instituted.

13.3 PREVENTION OF PPH

1. Having identified a high-risk feature either antenatally or during labour, an intravenous infusion of Hartmann's solution should be set up as soon as the woman is established in labour.
2. At the same time, blood is taken for haemoglobin estimation and serum is sent for cross-matching of two units of blood.
3. At delivery syntometrine (one ampoule) is given with the delivery of the anterior shoulder as usual.
4. In addition, an infusion of 20 i.u. syntocinon in 500 ml Hartmann's solution is commenced, to be infused at a rate of 40 drop min-1 for at least 1 h.

13.4 MANAGEMENT OF PPH

1. The uterus is massaged to encourage contraction. If this fails, medical help should be sought and 500 μg ergometrine can be given i.v. (this may cause the woman to vomit).
2. On arrival, the SHO should set up two intravenous lines:
   a. A syntocinon infusion of 20 i.u. syntocinon in 500 ml Hartmann's.
   b. Volume replacement in the form of crystalloid, or if the woman is clinically shocked a colloid, such as Haemaccel.
3. At the time of inserting the i.v. lines, blood will be taken for haemoglobin estimation and cross-matching of at least two units of blood.
4. Commence bimanual massage (Figure 13.1).
5. If the bleeding does not respond to these measures, the registrar should be called. Further bleeding in the presence of a well-contracted uterus should raise the suspicion of genital tract injury or retained placental fragments. This is an indication for careful inspection and examination of the genital tract.

13.4.1 Examination under anaesthesia

This may be provided by an epidural block if one is already *in situ*, or otherwise by general anaesthesia. A good light and at least one assistant are also required. The vagina and cervix are examined carefully for the presence of lacerations, and the uterine cavity is explored digitally, to detect retained placental fragments.

The cervix is explored for lacerations by means of three sponge-holding forceps (SHF). The *first* SHF is put on the cervix at 12 o'clock and the second is placed at 2 o'clock. The cervix between the SHFs is stretched and inspected for tears. The third

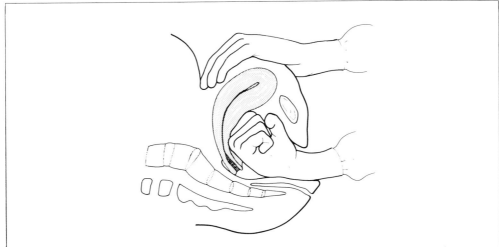

Figure 13.1   Bimanual compression of the uterus. The fist in the vagina forms a platform against which the fundus of the uterus can be massaged

SHF is then placed at 4 o'clock, and the cervix between the second and third pair is stretched and inspected. The *second* SHF is then moved to 6 o'clock and the cervix is inspected between the third and the second SHF. The process is repeated until the first SHF is encountered. In this way no lacerations will be missed.

If this examination is negative, then more senior medical help should be sought before the anaesthetic is reversed, and the prospect of laparotomy should be considered. This is to exclude uterine rupture, and to allow various specific surgical procedures to be performed in an attempt to control the haemorrhage (see below).

Inserting a pack within the uterine cavity is not a worthwhile procedure, since this will tend to prevent further contraction of the myometrium and thereby exacerbate the bleeding.

In the case of a placenta which is examined and found to be obviously missing a cotyledon, this will usually result in the need for evacuation of the uterus under anaesthetic before the woman leaves the labour ward.

13.5 MANAGEMENT OF MASSIVE PPH

This is defined as blood loss of an amount equivalent to the patient's circulating blood volume over a period of a few hours. For practical purposes the following measures should be considered when the patient has required transfusion of more than two units of blood.

1. Follow the measures as listed above.
2. Ensure that at least two i.v. lines are functioning. Large bore cannulae (at least 16 gauge) should be used.

3. Fluids are given to replace depleted intravascular volume:
   a. Up to 2 *l* of Hartmann's solution.
   b. Up to 3 units (1.5 *l*) Haemaccel.
   c. Uncross-matched blood of the patient's group.
   d. Cross-matched blood as soon as possible.
   e. O negative blood should be used only as a last resort.
      In an emergency situation the use of blood filters and blood warming devices is not recommended. However, pressurized infusion bags should be used.
      Stored blood becomes deficient in platelets and clotting factors therefore one unit of fresh frozen plasma (FFP) should be given for every 6 units of blood.
4. The anaesthetic registrar is called. The obstetric registrar and/or senior registrar should already be present.
5. The blood bank is informed, and a further 20 ml blood are sent for cross-matching. At least 6 units of blood should be requested.
6. The duty haematologist is informed of the clinical situation and of any associated clotting deficiency.
7. A central venous pressure line is inserted and a urinary catheter in order to be able to monitor fluid balance accurately.
8. During these events, one person should be allocated to measure and record the following at frequent intervals:
   a. Pulse rate (preferably via ECG monitor).
   b. Blood pressure.
   c. CVP.
   d. Hourly urine output.
   e. Drugs, including fluids, administered to the patient.
9. The obstetric consultant should be informed.
10. If bleeding continues and laparotomy is required, the following measures may be considered:
    a. Direct intramyometrial injection of 250 μg 15-methyl-prostaglandin $F_2\alpha$ in saline, repeat as often as necessary every 5–20 min.
    b. The broad ligament can be opened and the uterine arteries ligated on each side.
    c. The internal iliac arteries can be ligated.
    d. Hysterectomy.

Chapter 14

Coagulopathy

14.1 DEFINITION

Disseminated intravascular coagulation (DIC) is the phenomenon whereby widespread clotting, consumption of clotting factors and platelets and fibrin deposition results in a bleeding tendency. Haemorrhage and consequent hypovolaemia are often the cause of DIC. Once established, DIC will exacerbate haemorrhage and a vicious circle is created as shown in Figure 14.1.

DIC does not occur as a primary event; it is always secondary to certain triggering factors.

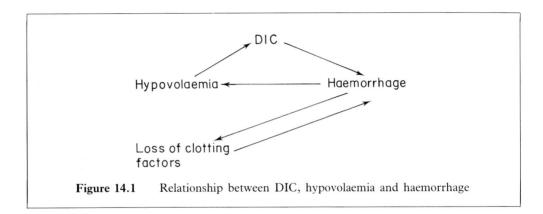

Figure 14.1 Relationship between DIC, hypovolaemia and haemorrhage

14.2   CAUSES

14.2.1   Obstetric causes of DIC

1. Placental abruption.
2. Amniotic fluid embolism.   } These conditions may result in *severe* DIC.
3. Eclampsia.
4. Pre-eclampsia.
5. Intra-uterine death.
6. Intra-uterine infection, including septic abortion.
7. Induced abortion with hypertonic fluids.
8. Large feto-maternal bleed.
9. Hydatidiform mole.
10. Placenta accreta.

14.2.2   Other causes

1. Hypovolaemia.
2. Septicaemia.
3. Incompatible blood transfusion.

DIC exhibits a wide spectrum of severity. In its least severe form, haemostasis is not impaired, but rapid progression to a severe form with haemostatic failure can occur unless the condition is recognized and dealt with appropriately.

14.3   LABORATORY FINDINGS IN DIC

1. Fibrin and fibrinogen degradation products (FDP) are increased. These result from increased fibrinolysis due to widespread fibrin deposition. FDPs can impair myometrial function.
2. Fibrinogen levels fall.
3. Platelets are reduced in number.
4. Factors V and VIII are reduced.

These factors will result in a prolongation of the *partial thromboplastin time*, which tests the intrinsic clotting system, the *prothrombin time*, which tests the extrinsic clotting system, and the *thrombin time*, which tests the final common pathway (see Figures 14.2 and 14.3).

In mild DIC with no bleeding tendency, the only finding may be slightly raised FDP levels. In severe DIC there will be profound thrombocytopaenia, gross depletion of clotting factors, particularly fibrinogen, and FDPs will be significantly raised.

14.4   MANAGEMENT OF A SUSPECTED COAGULOPATHY

This should be carried out in conjunction with a consultant haemotologist. The most important principle in the management of a patient with a clotting disorder

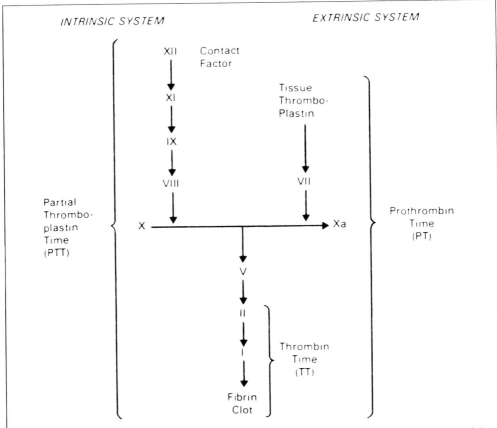

Figure 14.2   Summary of the intrinsic and extrinsic clotting systems. The partial thromboplastin time reflects the intrinsic system whilst the prothrombin time reflects the activity of the extrinsic system

is *to maintain her circulating volume*. This will prevent renal failure and encourage clearance of FDPs by the liver, as well as breaking the vicious circle of the DIC.

If the coagulopathy develops before delivery, the condition often resolves once delivery has occurred, provided hypovolaemia is avoided.

When a coagulopathy is suspected:

1. Unless already present, two intravenous lines are established with 16 gauge cannulae.
2. When siting the i.v. line, 15 ml blood are taken and divided as follows:
    a.   5 ml into EDTA tube for haemoglobin, haematocrit, and platelet count.
    b.   4.5 ml into citrated tube for estimation of:
        (i)   Partial thromboplastin time (PTT).
        (ii) Prothrombin time (PT).
        (iii) Thrombin time (TT).
        (iv) Fibrinogen level.

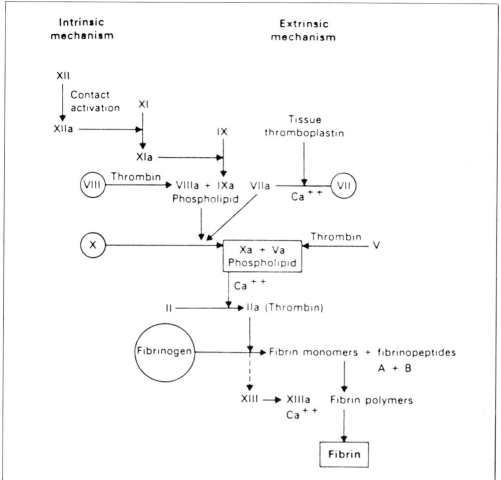

Figure 14.3   The clotting cascade. Activation via tissue thromboplastins (extrinsic mechanism) or contact activation from platelets (intrinsic mechanism) eventually results in the formation of fibrin from fibrinogen

c.   2.0 ml Into EACA tube for estimation of fibrin degradation products (FDP).
d.   Remainder into clotted tube for cross-matching of two units of blood.
These specimens should be dealt with urgently, but the results are *not* awaited before appropriate therapy is given.
3.   Fluid and volume replacement is commenced (see below).
4.   Meanwhile, two units of fresh frozen plasma (FFP) are placed in a 37 °C water bath to thaw.
5.   Measures to prevent further blood loss are instituted as in Chapters 12 and 13. If the coagulopathy occurs before delivery, vaginal delivery will create less demand on the clotting system than will Caesarean section, and therefore is to be preferred if possible. Measures should be taken to avoid soft tissue damage during delivery.

14.5 INTRAVENOUS THERAPY IN COAGULOPATHY

This includes (in order of importance):

1. Plasma volume replacement.
2. Replacement of clotting factors.
3. Replacement of red cells.

Initially, either crystalloid (e.g. Hartmann's solution) or artificial colloid (e.g. Haemaccel) can be infused. If crystalloid is used, two to three times the estimated blood loss should be infused, as it stays in the circulation for a shorter time than a colloid.

Dextran should be avoided since it interferes with platelet function and the interpretation of blood grouping and cross-matching tests. It is also associated with allergic anaphylactoid reactions.

Haemaccel (polygeline—a derivative of bovine gelatin) is probably the best choice for initial resuscitation since it does not have the disadvantages of dextran. Up to three units (1.5 ℓ) can be infused rapidly before blood is available.

Two units of FFP are given as soon as they are thawed. FFP contains all the coagulation factors present in the plasma of whole blood except platelets. Ideally the FFP should be of the same ABO and Rhesus group as the patient, but cross-matching is not necessary. This will provide the clotting factors which are deficient in stored banked blood. Uncross-matched whole blood of the same blood group as the patient should be given until cross-matched blood is available (this usually takes at least 40 min).

Fresh whole blood is no longer available in the UK because of hazards of transmission of hepatitis B and other infections, including cytomegalovirus, syphilis and AIDS.

The volume of blood transfused will depend on the amount of blood loss. The administration of fluids should be monitored by the presence of a central line and a urinary catheter. One unit of FFP should be given for every four to six units of banked blood, and calcium levels should be checked after every sixth unit of blood since citrate in stored blood complexes calcium. Fibrinogen concentrates and platelet transfusions are generally *not* indicated in DIC. Fibrinogen is present in adequate quantities in FFP, and concentrates carry risks of infections as above. Platelets are deficient in FFP and stored blood, but it is not usually necessary to give platelet transfusions to achieve haemostasis, unless the platelet count falls to rise and remains at an exceptionally low level of $<20 \times 10^9 \ \ell^{-1}$.

Chapter 15

Fetal Distress

15.1 INTRODUCTION

Fetal distress is defined as fetal acidosis resulting from a hypoxic insult. The hypoxia may be transitory, intermittent or continuous, and may result in abnormalities of the fetal heart rate tracing on cardiotocography. It is very unusual for fetal acidosis to co-exist with an entirely normal fetal heart rate tracing, but an abnormal tracing correlates poorly with the fetal acid–base status, and false positives occur frequently. For this reason facilities for measuring fetal scalp pH are a necessary back-up to cardiotocographic monitoring in labour.

15.2 ANTENATAL RISK FACTORS

Certain antenatal complications may lead to progressive fetal compromise and therefore a diminished capacity of the fetus to withstand the rigours of labour. These complications include:

1. Asymmetrical intra-uterine growth retardation.
2. Rhesus iso-immunization.

3. Maternal diabetes mellitus.
4. Pre-eclampsia and eclampsia.
5. Maternal sickle cell disease.
6. Recurrent antepartum haemorrhage.
7. Intra-uterine infection.
8. Chorio-amnionitis.

The degree to which the fetus is affected by these conditions can be assessed antenatally by fetal growth on ultrasound, fetal activity, amniotic fluid assessment on ultrasound, and cardiotocography. If the fetus is thought to be severely compromised antenatally, delivery by Caesarean section may be indicated, to avoid the added stress of labour.

15.3   INTRAPARTUM RISK FACTORS

The following intrapartum events can lead to fetal hypoxia:

1. Maternal hypotension.
    a. Supine hypotension.
    b. Hypovolaemia secondary to haemorrhage.
    c. Hypotensive drugs, including local anaesthetic drugs used for epidural top-ups.
2. Uterine hypertonus.
    a. From syntocinon overdose.
    b. Resulting from the inadvertent administration of a bolus of intravenous syntocinon.
3. Placental abruption.
4. Fetal bleeding, e.g. from vasa praevia (see Section 12.3.4).
5. Cord prolapse.
6. Uterine rupture.
7. Maternal cardio-respiratory arrest.
8. Prolonged labour.
9. Eclampsia.

These events may lead to fetal distress even when the preceding pregnancy has been entirely uncomplicated. The preterm fetus is particularly susceptible to acidosis in labour (see Chapter 9).

15.4   DIAGNOSIS

15.4.1   CTG abnormalities in labour

The abnormal CTG has been classified in several different ways, e.g. Type I and Type II decelerations, but many of these classifications do not help with clinical interpretation. We recommend that the CTG should be described, as this teaches the observer to analyse the CTG in some detail, and conveys more information when the tracing is being discussed between two people. Examples of the description will be found in the legends to the CTGs in this chapter.

The normal CTG is described in Chapter 2 (Section 2.4).

15.4.1.1   ABNORMALITIES OF VARIABILITY

Reduced baseline variability (BV)

Baseline variability is a very important feature of a normal CTG, and reduced variability has been shown to be associated with intra-uterine death, fetal acidosis and low Apgar scores.

Baseline variability can be assessed by considering the oscillatory frequency and oscillatory amplitude (see Figure 15.1). Oscillatory frequency is affected by FHR and as this increases by 10 beats min^{-1}, the oscillatory frequency falls by 1 cycle min^{-1}.

A tracing with an oscillatory amplitude of 3–5 beats min^{-1} but normal oscillatory frequency is less likely to be associated with fetal acidosis than when both parameters are reduced.

Causes of reduced baseline variability:

1.   Fetal hypoxia.
2.   Drugs:
    a.   Alcohol.
    b.   Opiates.
    c.   Pethidine.
    d.   Diazepam (see Figure 15.2).
    e.   Phenothiazines.
3.   Fetal sleep is associated with decreased BV of not longer than 30 min duration.

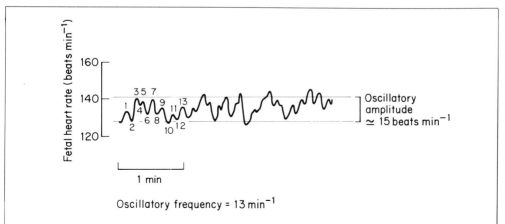

Figure 15.1   A diagram to illustrate oscillatory amplitude, which is the mean difference between maximum and minimum fetal heart rate, and the oscillatory frequency, which is the number of changes of direction of fetal heart rate per minute as shown

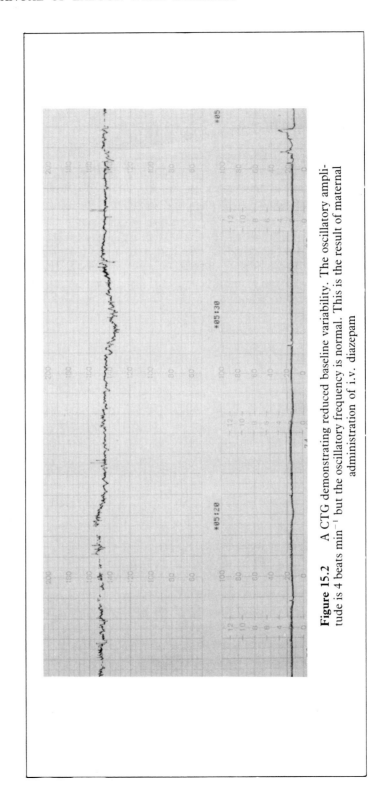

Figure 15.2   A CTG demonstrating reduced baseline variability. The oscillatory amplitude is 4 beats min^{-1} but the oscillatory frequency is normal. This is the result of maternal administration of i.v. diazepam

4. CNS abnormalities:
   a. Anencephaly.
   b. Microcephaly.

Baseline variability can be considered as a means of assessing fetal *reserve*, whereas decelerations of the FHR indicate the *mechanism* of the insult.
Management: A fetal blood sample (FBS) is indicated except in the following circumstances:

1. The reduced BV is due to the maternal administration of pethidine (or diazepam).
2. The period of reduced BV lasts less than 30 min.

Increased baseline variability

This particular CTG abnormality is usually called a sinusoidal pattern and is highly suggestive of fetal compromise and is associated with a 50–75 per cent perinatal mortality. It is seen in association with:

1. Severe fetal anaemia (e.g. due to Rhesus iso-immunization or bleeding from vasa praevia)
2. Hypoxia of the fetal myocardium

Thie pattern is characterized by increased variability of >15 beats min^{-1} and resembles a sine wave with a fixed periodicity of 2–5 cycles min^{-1}.
It has been classified as

1. Minor: variability of 15–30 beats min^{-1} (Figure 15.3).
2. Marked: variability of more than 30 beats min^{-1} (Figure 15.4).

The greater the oscillatory amplitude, the lower the fetal scalp pH.
Management: This CTG abnormality should prompt a FBS and estimation of fetal haematocrit.

15.4.1.2 BASELINE ABNORMALITIES

Baseline tachycardia

1. Moderate: 160–180 beats min^{-1} (Figure 15.5).
2. Severe: more than 180 beats min^{-1}.
   Factors associated with moderate fetal tachycardia:
   a. Maternal cardiac failure.
   b. Maternal thyrotoxiccosis.
   c. Extreme fetal prematurity (as the autonomic nervous system matures, vagal slowing of the basal heart rate becomes apparent).
   Factors associated with severe fetal tachycardia:
   a. Fetal hypoxia.
   b. Maternal or fetal infection with or without pyrexia.

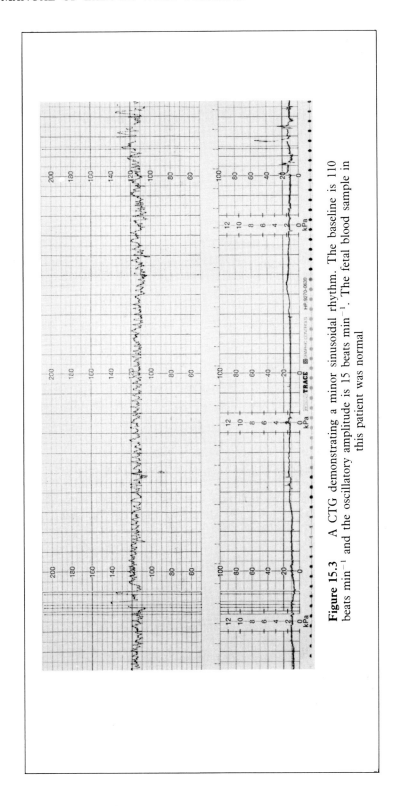

Figure 15.3 A CTG demonstrating a minor sinusoidal rhythm. The baseline is 110 beats min^{-1} and the oscillatory amplitude is 15 beats min^{-1}. The fetal blood sample in this patient was normal

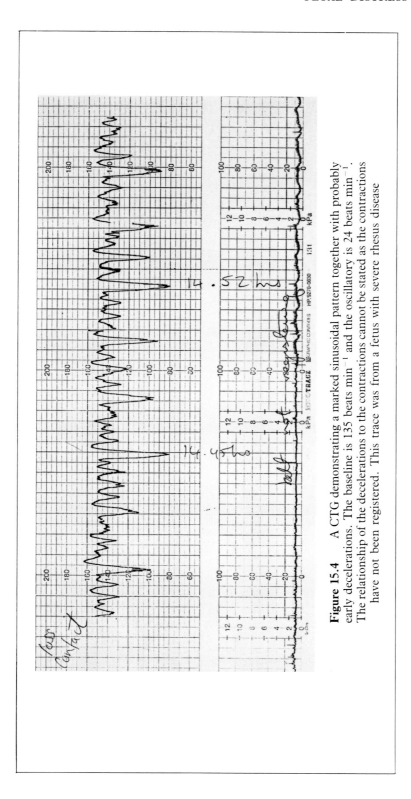

Figure 15.4   A CTG demonstrating a marked sinusoidal pattern together with probably early decelerations. The baseline is 135 beats min^{-1} and the oscillatory is 24 beats min^{-1}. The relationship of the decelerations to the contractions cannot be stated as the contractions have not been registered. This trace was from a fetus with severe rhesus disease

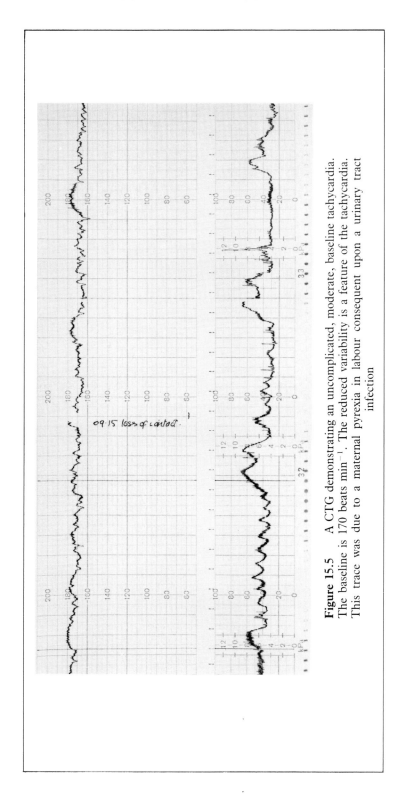

Figure 15.5   A CTG demonstrating an uncomplicated, moderate, baseline tachycardia. The baseline is 170 beats min⁻¹. The reduced variability is a feature of the tachycardia. This trace was due to a maternal pyrexia in labour consequent upon a urinary tract infection

c. Maternally administered drugs, e.g. β-sympathomimetics, hydralazine, adrenaline, atropine.

Baseline bradycardia

1. Moderate: 100–120 beats min^{-1} (Figure 15.6). A moderate baseline bradycardia with good baseline variability and no decelerations is usually inocuous.
2. Severe: less than 100 beats min^{-1}.
   Severe fetal bradycardia may be due to:
   a. Fetal cardiac dysrrhythmias and cardiac anomalies.
   b. Maternally administered drugs, e.g. local anaesthetics, nicotine, digoxin, morphine.
   c. Fetal haemorrhage.
   d. Fetal hypoxia.
   A severe fetal bradycardia or tachycardia should be investigated further by fetal scalp pH determinations.

15.4.1.3 DECELERATIONS

Single deceleration

A single isolated fetal heart deceleration (Figure 15.7), particularly if it can be related to a specific event, such as supine hypotension, or following rupture of the membranes and which subsequently returns to a normal pattern requires no specific action.

Persistent decelerations

These may be classified as:

1. Early decelerations. An early deceleration occurs during a contraction and is over by the time the contraction is over. It is usually V-shaped, and appears as the mirror-image of the uterine contraction. It results from stimulation of the vagus nerve, is most commonly due to head compression, and does not usually represent fetal distress. Recurrent deep decelerations, however, may be associated with fetal acidosis, particularly in the preterm infant.
2. Late decelerations. The deceleration begins after the beginning of the contraction, and recovery occurs after the contraction finishes. The deceleration is U-shaped (see Figure 15.8).
   Less favourable features of these decelerations include:
   a. Loss of character of the fetal heart trace (i.e. the trace has little variability during the deceleration and appears as a solid line).
   b. Asymmetry of the deceleration, when recovery of the fetal heart rate to the baseline occurs over several minutes.
   c. Increasing lag time between the peak of the contraction and the lowest point of the FHR deceleration. Decelerations with a lag time of more than 18 s are of serious significance.
   d. There is a weak positive correlation between the amplitude of decelerations and fetal asphyxia.

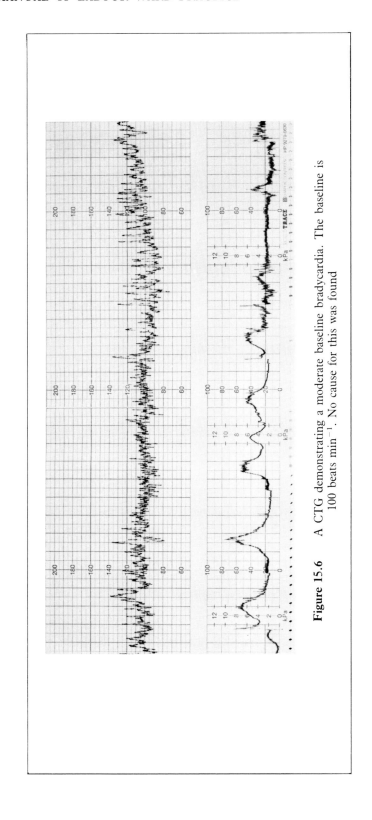

Figure 15.6   A CTG demonstrating a moderate baseline bradycardia. The baseline is 100 beats min^{-1}. No cause for this was found

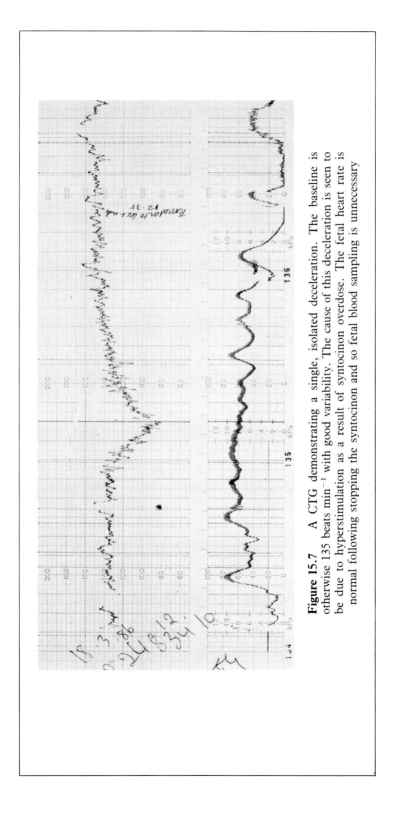

Figure 15.7 A CTG demonstrating a single, isolated deceleration. The baseline is otherwise 135 beats min^{-1} with good variability. The cause of this deceleration is seen to be due to hyperstimulation as a result of syntocinon overdose. The fetal heart rate is normal following stopping the syntocinon and so fetal blood sampling is unnecessary

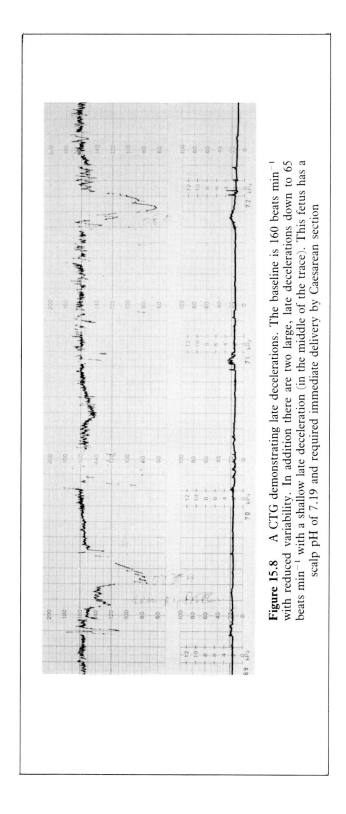

Figure 15.8   A CTG demonstrating late decelerations. The baseline is 160 beats min^{-1} with reduced variability. In addition there are two large, late decelerations down to 65 beats min^{-1} with a shallow late deceleration (in the middle of the trace). This fetus has a scalp pH of 7.19 and required immediate delivery by Caesarean section

Late decelerations are commonly associated with fetal myocardial hypoxia, and should always be further investigated (see below) with a fetal scalp pH.

3. Variable decelerations. Variable decelerations have no consistent relationship to uterine contractions and are often of different shapes and amplitudes (Figure 15.9.

   These may be associated with umbilical cord compression or fetal hypoxia and should always be investigated further (see below) with a fetal scalp pH.

4. Complicated patterns. Any combination of the abnormalities of fetal heart listed above constitute a complicated pattern. A complicated pattern, e.g. reduced baseline variability with a severe fetal tachycardia, is of more ominous significance than each abnormality considered in isolation, that is, it is more likely to be associated with fetal hypoxia.

   Examples of complicated patterns are shown in Section 13.9.

   Summary. The most worrying features of a CTG trace are decelerations associated with contractions, particularly if they are of delayed onset, or are associated with reduced baseline variability or a baseline tachycardia. If the CTG trace shows no change of the fetal heart with contractions and good baseline variability, then, regardless of the baseline FHR, it is reasonably certain that the fetus is not asphyxiated.

15.4.2   Meconium staining of the amniotic fluid

Meconium is faecal staining of the amniotic fluid and occurs in response to vagal stimulation. This depends upon the maturity of the fetal autonomic nervous system and therefore meconium-staining is uncommon before 34 weeks gestation. Conversely up to 30 per cent post-term fetuses will pass meconium in labour. During a breech delivery the passage of meconium is to be expected as the breech passes through the maternal pelvis.

Meconium is more likely to be associated with fetal hypoxia when:

1. It occurs early in labour.
2. The meconium is thick in consistency and pea green in colour (i.e. fresh). Old, dark brown meconium is less likely to be associated with hypoxia but may still produce the meconium aspiration syndrome.
3. It is associated with CTG abnormalities.

In each of these instances, a fetal scalp pH is advised (see below).

In the presence of meconium, particular care should be taken to clear the pharynx of the neonate immediately after delivery to prevent the meconium aspiration syndrome. This baby's mouth should *always* be aspirated first as nasal aspiration causes the baby to gasp (see Chapter 6).

15.5   FETAL BLOOD SAMPLING

Fetal distress is confirmed by the finding of a low fetal scalp pH in the presence of CTG abnormalities and/or meconium staining of the amniotic fluid.

Fetal blood sampling (FBS) is indicated in the following instances:

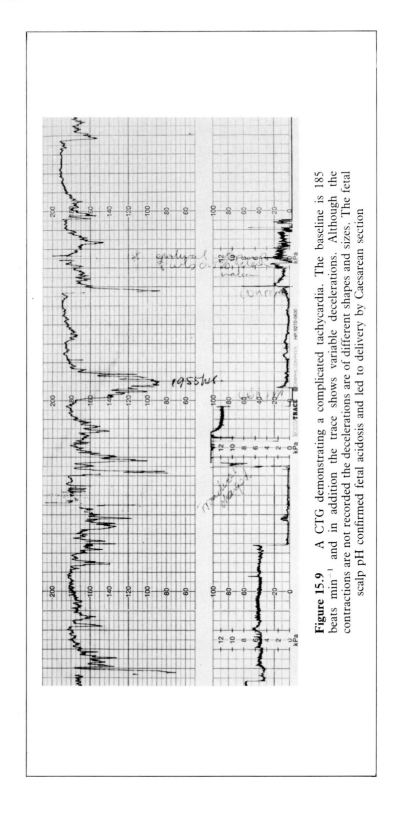

Figure 15.9   A CTG demonstrating a complicated tachycardia. The baseline is 185 beats min^{-1} and in addition the trace shows variable decelerations. Although the contractions are not recorded the decelerations are of different shapes and sizes. The fetal scalp pH confirmed fetal acidosis and led to delivery by Caesarean section

1. Meconium staining of the amniotic fluid early in labour or that develops in labour.
2. Meconium staining of the amniotic fluid and an abnormal CTG (including loss of baseline variability).
3. CTG abnormalities:
    a. Persistent severe fetal bradycardia or severe fetal tachycardia.
    b. Persistent late decelerations.
    c. Persistent variable decelerations.
    d. Complicated pattern.
    e. Marked sinusoidal pattern.
    f. Persistent loss of baseline variability in the absence of an obvious cause.

The fetal scalp pH gives information about the acid–base status of the fetus at the moment in time when it was performed. It does not predict fetal acid–base status at delivery. Therefore, when the indications persist the FBS should be repeated at least every 60 min until delivery.

When the indication for a FBS occurs in the second stage, the fetal scalp pH will assist in the decision as to whether delivery is necessary immediately, or whether it is appropriate to await further descent and rotation of the fetal head and spontaneous delivery.

15.5.1   Technique

This technique is easily learnt and the procedure usually takes about 5–10 min. Figure 15.10 illustrates the necessary equipment.

1. The patient is placed in the left lateral position with her hips and knees flexed and with an assistant supporting the uppermost leg. Alternatively the lithotomy position can be used, provided a pillow is put under one buttock to avoid supine hypotension which may produce a falsely low pH.
2. The vulva is cleaned and a vaginal examination is performed in the usual way. The appropriate size amnioscope is selected. It is introduced downwards and backwards into the vagina with the obturator in place. The obturator is then removed and the fibre-optic light is attached. The amnioscope is held such that a tight seal is formed on the fetal head. Amniotic fluid, meconium, mucus and blood are wiped meticulously away from the fetal head by means of cotton wool balls, held in sponge-holding forceps.
3. The fetal head is sprayed by an assistant with ethyl chloride. This quickly evaporates causing a reactive hyperaemia. The head should then be covered with sterile paraffin grease applied by means of a dental swab in a holder. This allows the blood to collect in drops.
4. The scalp is punctured by firm pressure with the guarded blade mounted in a holder (see Figure 15.11). Free flowing blood is collected into a heparinized tube either by capillary action or by gentle suction at the other end. The aim is to obtain a complete column of blood, at least 5 cm in length, with little or no air bubbles. Up to 10 per cent of air bubbles are acceptable.
5. The heparinized tube full of blood should be handed to an assistant. Clotting of the sample is prevented by inserting a small metal rod about 1 cm long into the

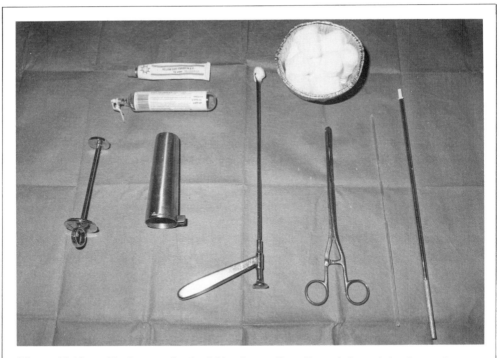

Figure 15.10   Equipment for fetal blood sampling. From left to right the equipment is the obturator and amnioscope, a swab for cleaning the fetal head, a pair of sponge holding forceps, a heparinized capillary tube and a guarded blade for making the incision in the fetal head. At the top of the picture is the ethyl chloride spray above which is the soft yellow paraffin grease

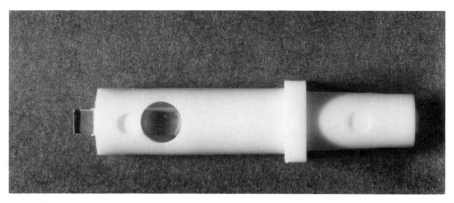

Figure 15.11   The guarded blade from the fetal blood sampling set. The amount of blade visible is 1.5 mm

capillary tube and agitating the blood by stroking a magnet up and down the outside of the tube.

6. A second sample should be taken into a separate tube.
7. Both specimens are measured on a pH meter immediately. If a print out is available it should be placed in the notes securely and labelled appropriately.

15.5.2 Interpretation of results

The pH is interpreted with the base deficit, since a low pH in the presence of a normal base deficit may imply that the fetus has been able to buffer the excess lactate produced as a result of anaerobic glycolysis. If lactic acid production continues, as a result of hypoxia, glycogenolysis will be reduced. This results in reduced cellular glucose availability for energy production and therefore asphyxia.

1. A pH or more than 7.25 is normal. (Base deficit of less than 8.0.)
2. A pH of 7.20–7.25 implies pre-asphyxia. (Base deficit of 8.0–12.0.)
3. A pH less than 7.20 implies asphyxia. (Base deficit of more than 12.0.)

If the FBS indicates asphyxia the baby should be delivered immediately.

If the FBS is normal but the CTG abnormality persists the FBS should be repeated every hour. The fetal scalp pH may be normal because the hypoxia is intermittent and buffered by the fetus.

If the FBS indicates pre-asphyxia management depends on the stage of labour:

1. In the first stage of labour, the FBS should be repeated after 30 min, if the CTG abnormality persists.
2. In the second stage of labour, pre-asphyxia should be treated by forceps or Ventouse delivery provided the relevant criteria apply (see Chapter 26). If the head is too high for safe delivery, Caesarean section should be performed.

15.6 COMMON PROBLEMS WITH FETAL SCALP pH ESTIMATION

1. Contamination of the sample with maternal blood or liquor will lead to erroneous results (amniotic fluid is alkaline and maternal blood may be acidic). This is avoided by ensuring that only a clean and uncontaminated sample is used.
2. Excessive caput succedaneum formation of the fetal head may lead to a falsely low pH.
3. Obtaining an uncontaminated sample may be difficult if the fetus has thick, long hair, which may be soaked in liquor or meconium. Occasionally the fetal hair must be cut with long-handled scissors to provide a clean, bare patch to be used for FBS.
4. If the fetal head is not fixed in the pelvis, then pressure with the guarded blade may push the head away from the amnioscope, causing amniotic fluid to obscure the field. An assistant providing pressure on the uterine fundus may prevent this.
5. The procedure can be difficult for the operator, particularly if the cervix is only

2–3 cm dilated, but with sufficient experience and patience, a sample can usually be obtained.
6. The procedure can be uncomfortable for the patient. Appropriate analgesia, particularly epidural block, will usually allow the operator to proceed.
7. The fetal scalp pH may not truly reflect the fetal condition in the presence of intra-uterine infection or placental abruption.

15.7 MANAGEMENT OF SUSPECTED FETAL DISTRESS

1. If syntocinon is being administered, the infusion should be stopped.
2. The patient should be turned onto her left side and given oxygen by face mask at $4 \; \ell \; min^{-1}$.
3. The maternal pulse rate and blood pressure should be taken and recorded.
4. A possible cause for the CTG abnormality should be sought.
5. If the CTG does not immediately improve, a vaginal examination should be performed to exclude a cord prolapse. Subsequent management will depend upon the cervical dilatation:
   a. Cervix less than 2 cm dilated. If the CTG abnormality is severe and there is no obvious cause then delivery by Caesarean section should be strongly considered as FBS is usually impossible.
   b. Cervix 2–9 cm dilated. A FBS should be performed and the patient managed according to the result (see above).
   c. Cervix fully dilated (10 cm). A FBS should be performed and the patient managed as above. This allows optimum management and will often avoid an instrumental delivery. If the CTG abnormality is serious, however, and the fetal head is in the outlet a forceps delivery is indicated.
6. Adequate paediatric support should be provided at the time of delivery. Cord pH determination is useful to confirm the diagnosis of fetal distress and may assist in paediatric management.

Chapter 16
Collapse

16.1 INTRODUCTION

Most obstetric patients are healthy and so if a patient collapses in labour or immediately after delivery, management may not be ideal unless some prior thought has been given to the situation. This chapter will provide guidelines on diagnosis and management.

Table 16.1   Causes of collapse at or immediately after delivery

Circulatory failure
1. Massive blood loss from:
    a.   Placental abruption.
    b.   Placenta praevia.
    c.   Genital tract injuries, including ruptured uterus.
    d.   Atonic uterus.
2. Septicaemic shock.
3. Acute uterine inversion.
4. Myocardial failure.
    a.   Pre-existing cardiac disease.
    b.   Myocardial infarction.
    c.   Cardiomyopathy of pregnancy.

Respiratory compromise
1. Amniotic fluid embolism
2. Pulmonary embolism
3. Pulmonary oedema
4. Aspiration (Mendelson's syndrome)

Intracranial pathology
1. Eclampsia
2. Epilepsy
3. Cerebral vascular accident
4. Subarachnoid haemorrhage
5. Acute withdrawal in drug abusers

Metabolic disturbances
1. Hypoglycaemia
2. Keto-acidotic coma
3. Water intoxication
4. Acute withdrawal from steroids
5. Acute hepatic failure
6. Anaphylaxis

Table 16.1 lists the causes of collapse.

16.2   MANAGEMENT

1. Ensure that the patient has a clear airway. If there is doubt insert an airway and give oxygen at 4 ℓ min^{-1} via a face mask.
2. Measure pulse rate and blood pressure.
3. Start an intravenous infusion of Hartmann's solution via a 16 gauge cannula. At the same time send venous blood for:
    a.   Haemoglobin estimation.
    b.   Group and save serum.
    c.   Urea and electrolytes.
    d.   Blood glucose.
    e.   Blood culture.

    f.   Clotting studies.

    g.   Arterial blood gases if the patient is cyanosed.

4.   Take a rapid history from anyone who observed the collapse and in particular ask:

    a.   Did the patient have a fit?

    b.   Did the patient complain of pain prior to collapse; if so, where was the pain?

    c.   Has the patient delivered the baby and the placenta?

    d.   Was the blood loss at delivery excessive?

    e.   Does the patient have a relevant medical history, for example, is she a known epileptic or a diabetic?

    f.   Was the patient known to be on any medication prior to the collapse or is she a known drug abuser?

5.   Make a thorough physical examination.

    a.   Look at the visible blood loss and make an estimate as to whether it is responsible for the collapse.

    b.   Is the patient shocked?

        (i)   A patient with tachycardia, low blood pressure and cold extremities is shocked and needs intravenous volume replacement urgently.

        (ii)   A patient with tachycardia, low blood pressure and warm extremities probably has a gram negative septicaemia.

        (iii)   A patient with low blood pressure and bradycardia may have raised intracranial pressure—check the pupils to see if they are even.

    c.   Examine the chest.

        (i)   Is there a pleural rub caused by a pulmonary embolism?

        (ii)   Is the JVP raised with basal crepitations because of pulmonary oedema?

        (iii)   Are there signs of inhaled vomitus?

        (iv)   Is there pink frothy sputum suggesting an amniotic fluid embolism?

    d.   Examine the abdomen.

        (i)   Is the abdomen rigid suggesting a uterine rupture?

        (ii)   If the baby is not delivered is the uterus woody hard due to placental abruption.

        (iii)   If the baby is delivered is the uterine fundus high and poorly contracted?

        (iv)   Is the uterine fundus deviated to one side suggesting a broad ligament haematoma?

        (v)   Is the uterine fundus impalpable because of an acute uterine inversion?

    e.   Perform a vaginal examination.

        (i)   Is there a large para-vaginal haematoma?

        (ii)   Is there a partial uterine inversion?

        (iii)   Are there obvious injuries to the lower genital tract?

16.3 MANAGEMENT OF CIRCULATORY FAILURE

16.3.1 Restore circulating volume

1.   Insert two large bore cannulae. These must be at least 16 gauge as blood cannot be forced rapidly through smaller cannulae.

2.   Give 2 ℓ of Hartmann's solution rapidly.

3. Monitor maternal pulse and blood pressure every 10 min.
4. If the systolic blood pressure is still less than 100 mmHg give up to 1.5 ℓ of Haemaccel.
5. If further fluids are still needed then blood should be given. Blood transfusion is indicated when:
   a. A third of calculated blood volume has been lost (see Table 16.2).
   b. The PCV is less than 30 per cent.

Table 16.2 Clinical estimation of percentage blood loss

Loss of total volume (%)	State of shock	Systolic blood pressure (mmHg)	Signs and symptoms
10–15	Compensated	120	Palpitations, dizziness, tachycardia
15–25	Mild	110	Thirst, sweating
25–35	Moderate	70–80	Restless, pallor, oliguria
35–40	Severe	50–70	Cyanosis, collapse
>40	Profound	<50	Air hunger, anuria

16.3.2 Stop the bleeding

1. Antepartum haemorrhage (see Chapter 12).
2. Postpartum haemorrhage (see Chapter 13).
3. Genital tract injury (see Chapter 25).
4. Abnormal coagulation (see Chapter 14).

16.4 SEPTICAEMIC SHOCK

The mortality rate for shock associated with sepsis in the non-pregnant population is about 50 per cent but survival in pregnancy is greater because patients are generally young and fit prior to the event. The bacteria involved may be *Escherichia coli*, enterococci, β-haemolytic streptococci, *Bacteroides* and *Clostridia*. The commonest situation resulting in septicaemia is after a Caesarean section in the presence of chorioamnionitis, but also after catheterization in women with urinary tract infections.

16.4.1 Diagnosis

Table 16.3 indicates the clinical signs.
   In addition to these signs patients with septicaemic shock may deteriorate during anaesthesia or fail to regain consciousness.

Table 16.3   Clinical signs of septicaemic shock

Sign	Early	Late
Mental state	Confused, restless	Coma
Extremities	Warm, sweaty	Cold
Cyanosis	None	Peripheral, central
Respiratory rate	Tachypnoea	Tachypnoea
Pulse rate (beats min^{-1})	<110	>110
Systolic pressure (mmHg)	> 80	< 80
Jaundice	Mild	Moderate
Coagulation defects	No	Yes

16.4.2   Investigations

1. Haemoglobin and white cell count.
2. Urea, electrolytes and creatinine.
3. Blood gases.
4. Blood culture.
5. MSU, high vaginal swab.

16.4.3   Management

1. Administer oxygen via a face mask at 4 l min^{-1}. If the patient is unable to maintain her airway or if the PaO$_2$ is less than 60 mmHg (8.0 kPa) intubation and assisted ventilation should be considered.
2. Correct circulating volume. This must be done under CVP control because it is easily possible to overload the patient in the early stages of the disease. A CVP reading of less than 4 cm water (measured at the sternal angle) suggest hypovolaemia which is best corrected with either fresh frozen plasma (FFP) or plasma protein fraction (PPF). This should be infused until the systolic blood pressure is over 100 mmHg and the urine output is more than 30 ml h^{-1}. If this fails or if the patient has an initial high CVP reading further fluid loading is contraindicated until the pulmonary artery wedge pressure is known (see Section 11.11).
3. When the patient is stable she should be transferred to an intensive care unit as detailed monitoring will be necessary.
4. If pulmonary artery wedge pressure measurements are not readily available and the patient has not responded to the above measures give 2 g of methylprednisolone intravenously once only. This is thought to act by preventing peripheral vasoconstriction and limiting the entry of bacterial toxins into cells.
5. Start antibiotics. Note that antibiotics should not be started until the above measures have been performed and appropriate cultures have been taken. Give broad spectrum antibiotic cover such as ampicillin 500 mg iv every 6 h and gentamicin 120 mg statim and then 80 mg every 8 h together with 500 mg of metronidazole iv every 6 h. Gentamicin levels should be monitored.

The toxic shock syndrome is due to staphylococcus and in this situation the blood cultures are negative and unless appropriate material (high vaginal swab and/ or products of conception) is gram stained the diagnosis will be missed. Treatment is by means of flucloxacillin and fucidin.
6.   Look for and manage the associated disseminated coagulopathy (see Chapter 14).

16.5   AMNIOTIC FLUID EMBOLISM

Amniotic fluid embolism is rare, occurring in about one in 30 000 live births but it carries a maternal mortality of about 80 per cent. The diagnosis is confirmed by finding fetal squamous cells or meconium in blood aspirated from the right side of the heart or in the lungs.

16.5.1   Pathophysiology

The means by which amniotic fluid enters the maternal circulation is unknown but is probably a result of premature placental separation which commonly coexists. The particulate matter in the amniotic fluid blocks the distal pulmonary artery tree. The acute pulmonary hypertension that results causes constriction of the pulmonary and coronary arteries via the vagus nerve leading to right heart failure. In addition the amniotic fluid causes a coagulopathy and hypofibrinogenaemia.

16.5.2   Predisposing factors

1.   ARM/SRM occurring at the height of a tumultuous contraction.
2.   Hypertonic uterine activity due to syntocinon stimulation with intact membranes.
3.   Labour following intra-uterine death.
4.   Intrapartum placental abruption.

16.5.3   Diagnosis

Amniotic fluid embolism may present:

1.   As sudden cardiac arrest usually preceded by a short period of respiratory distress. Even with vigorous resuscitation these patients have a poor prognosis.
2.   Gradually with the following signs and symptoms:
     a.   Dyspnoea, cyanosis, tachypnoea.
     b.   Shock.
     c.   Undue maternal anxiety and feelings of doom.
     d.   Unexplained vaginal bleeding.
     e.   Grand mal convulsions.

16.5.4   Management

Survival is possible but only if the diagnosis is suspected and vigorous treatment is begun early. Therefore on suspicion of an amniotic embolism:

1. Give 100 per cent oxygen initially via face mask.
2. Start an infusion of normal saline and send blood for:
   a. Haemoglobin and cross-matching, four units.
   b. Clotting studies.
   c. Blood gases.
   d. Urea and electrolytes.
   e. Blood glucose.
   f. Blood culture.
3. Insert a CVP line and organize a portable chest X-ray.
4. If PaO_2 <80 mmHg (9.3 kPa) on 100 per cent oxygen the patient will need to be intubated and positive pressure ventilation commenced.
5. If the CVP is <8 cm water (measured at the sternal angle) fluid replacement should be commenced, preferably with fresh frozen plasma (FFP) until this CVP is achieved. If the CVP is >8 cm water a Swan–Ganz thermodilution catheter should be inserted to measure cardiac output particularly if the patient is also hypotensive (systolic blood pressure of <90 mmHg). If this is required send blood from the right side of the heart to be stained for fetal squamous cells in order to confirm the diagnosis.
6. If the fibrinogen titre is <1/64 or in the absence of this test if the thrombin or prothrombin times are prolonged give 2 units of FFP. Further management of the coagulopathy is given in Chapter 14.
7. Start intravenous cephradine 500 mg every 6 h and metronidazole 500 mg every 8 h.
8. Deliver the baby, preferably vaginally to avoid the added risks of general anaesthesia.

16.6 PULMONARY EMBOLISM

Most pulmonary emboli in pregnancy occur during labour or in the immediate puerperium. For the past 20 years thromboembolism has been a leading cause of maternal death.

16.6.1 Prophylaxis

The immediate puerperium is the time of maximum risk of thromboembolism for all mothers. This is because of:

1. An increase in absolute levels of clotting factors occurs in pregnancy.
2. Venous stasis and compression of the pelvic veins.
3. The decrease in plasma volume that occurs immediately following delivery.

General measures to prevent thromboemboli include adequate hydration in labour together with early mobilization.

Hospitals differ on their policies for patients undergoing Caesarean section:

1. Early mobilization only.
2. Graduated ambulatory support stockings fitted prior to operation.

3.   The intra-operative use of inflatable leg bags.
4.   Prophylactic subcutaneous heparin.

16.6.2   Presentation

1.   Large pulmonary emboli present with pleuritic pain, blood stained sputum and breathlessness.
2.   Smaller emboli may present with breathlessness alone.
3.   There may be a preceding DVT.

16.6.3   Investigations

1.   Chest X-ray. Unless there is pulmonary infarction this is rarely diagnostic but helps exclude other pathologies. It is a necessary pre-requisite to a ventilation-perfusion scan.
2.   ECG. Right heart strain may be manifest as an S wave in lead I and a Q wave with T wave inversion in lead III. However, these changes may also be seen in late normal pregnancy.
3.   Blood gases. Hypoxia with a P_{O_2} of <80 mmHg (9.3 kPa) is strongly suggestive of a pulmonary embolism.
4.   Ventilation-perfusion scan. This is a radio-isotope lung scan and will demonstrate areas of under-perfusion consequent upon the pulmonary embolism. It should be regarded as diagnostic.

16.6.4   Management

1.   As soon as the diagnosis is suspected commence a continuous intravenous infusion of heparin providing 40 000 units per day.
2.   If the diagnosis is confirmed check that there is optimal anticoagulation by means of a heparin assay or a thrombin clotting time. Heparin levels of 0.3–5.0 units per ml or a thrombin time of two and a half times the control, should be achieved.
3.   If the patient has delivered, give ten days of intravenous heparin and then change to oral warfarin therapy. Breast feeding is not contraindicated.
4.   If the patient has not delivered, the ten day course of intravenous heparin is followed by 5000–7500 units every 12 h, subcutaneously, continuing until six weeks after delivery. Do *not* stop the subcutaneous heparin for labour or Caesarean section. Subcutaneous heparin may be monitored by means of anti-factor X_a activity which should be between 0.05–0.15 units.
5.   *Massive pulmonary embolism* usually results in systemic hypotension with right ventricular failure. The advice of a cardiothoracic surgeon should be sought with a view to performing a pulmonary embolectomy. Perinatal mortality is high following the procedure.
6.   *Recurrent pulmonary emboli*, despite full dose heparin, require the assistance of an expert haematologist and a vascular surgeon. If such help is not available streptokinase may be given at an empirical dose of 600 000 units statim followed by 100 000 units hourly for 72 h.
7.   The combined oral contraceptive pill is contraindicated in all patients with a history of thromboembolism.

16.7   PULMONARY ASPIRATION SYNDROME

Measures taken to prevent pulmonary aspiration syndrome (Mendelson's syndrome) are described in Section 3.8. The syndrome occurs when acid stomach contents (with a pH of less than 3.5) are aspirated into the bronchial tree. The acid contents cause a chemical pneumonitis with oedema, destruction of the endotracheal lining, transudation and capillary destruction. Finally there is necrosis of lung tissue.

16.7.1   Diagnosis

1. Commonly the aspiration is observed.
2. Initially there is intense bronchoconstriction followed by a reduction in perfusion leading to hypoxaemia and severe metabolic acidosis.
3. The chest X-ray initially may show a 'white-out' which may be generalized or localized to a major lung segment. Later there are changes of pulmonary oedema (Figure 11.3).

16.7.2   Immediate treatment

1. Aspirate the oro-pharynx and test its pH. If the pH is more than 3.5 the subsequent course is usually benign. If the pH is less than 3.5 the mortality is up to 25 per cent.
2. Intubate the patient and ventilate with 100 per cent oxygen using a low dose of volatile anaesthetic agent to complete the operation.
3. *Do not* attempt to wash out the bronchi or instill sodium bicarbonate as this will aggravate the situation.
4. If the pH is less than 3.5 give 1 g methylprednisolone i.v. followed by 100 mg hydrocortisone i.v. every 6 h for 48 h.

16.7.3   Long term management

1. Transfer the patient to ITU.
2. Continue ventilation for at least 6 h to maintain the P_{O_2} at more than 60 mmHg (8.0 kPa).
3. If bronchospasm is present give aminophylline 250 mg intravenously slowly.
4. Correct the metabolic acidosis.
5. Start intensive chest physiotherapy.
6. Strict fluid balance is essential.
7. Monitor serum albumin, and replace if serum levels are less than 25 g ℓ^{-1}. Albumin is lost in the pulmonary transudate.
8. In severe cases pulmonary artery wedge pressure measurements are vital. Over-transfusion or the injudicious use of colloids may superimpose the condition of 'wet lung'.
9. Long term outlook cannot be predicted.

Chapter 17

Retained Placenta

17.1 INTRODUCTION

A retained placenta is usually diagnosed if the placenta is undelivered 30 min after delivery of the infant.

17.1.1 Causes

1. The placenta is still wholly or partially attached.
2. An hour glass constriction of the lower segment, usually the result of ergometrine.
3. Pathological adherence of the placenta.

17.2 TREATMENT

1. The bladder is emptied by catheterization.
2. If the cord is still attached 30 min may be allowed to elapse after the syntometrine has been given and then a further attempt at controlled cord traction can take place (see Section 1.9). This will be successful if the retained placenta was due to an hour glass constriction of the lower segment because the effect of the ergometrine (contained in the syntometrine) will now have worn off.
3. If this fails or the cord has snapped a manual removal of the placenta is usually necessary, which will require good analgesia.

Note: Do not handle the uterus or attempt Credé's manoeuvre of squeezing the fundus as you will provoke severe bleeding if the placenta is still partially attached.

17.2.1   Manual removal of the placenta

1. An infusion of normal saline is commenced after insertion of a cannula of at least 16 gauge.
2. Blood is taken at the same time for haemoglobin estimation and for two units of blood to be cross-matched.
3. Good analgesia is achieved. This means either an epidural or spinal anaesthetic or a general anaesthetic. If a general anaesthetic is administered the same precautions should be taken as it the patient was in labour (see Section 3.8) as the risks of inhalation of stomach contents are still present.
4. Figure 17.1 illustrates the method of removing the placenta. The patient is placed in the lithotomy position; cleansed, draped with sterile towels and the bladder is catheterized. The operator's left hand controls the fundus of the uterus through the maternal abdominal wall. The right hand is well lubricated with Hibitane cream and passed into the uterus. Taking a fold of membranes the placenta is sheared off the uterine wall such that it comes to lie along the operator's hand and wrist and can be removed. The placenta must not be detached by a scraping action of the fingers as this may perforate the uterus.
5. Antibiotics do not need to be given prophylactically.

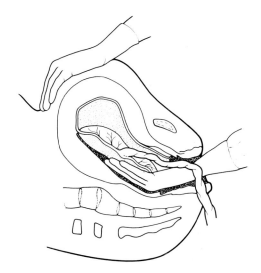

Figure 17.1   The method of manual removal of the placenta. The operator's left hand controls the uterine fundus through the maternal abdomen. The right hand is then inserted through the cervix and the placenta is detached from the uterus. When the placenta lies in the operator's hand it is removed

17.3 MORBIDLY ADHERENT PLACENTA

The entire placenta or just a small part may be morbidly adherent. The condition is usually only recognized when it is difficult to separate the placenta at manual removal. The subsequent haemorrhage usually necessitates hysterectomy but fortunately the condition is very rare.

If the placenta cannot be easily separated at the time of manual removal it may be morbidly adherent. If bleeding does not ensue the placenta should be left in the uterus and allowed to slough off.

Chapter 18
Twin Delivery

18.1   INTRODUCTION AND RISKS

The incidence of twins is about 1 in 80 deliveries but has a wide geographical variation. Twin pregnancy carries significantly increased risks of the following *antenatal* complications:

1. Spontaneous abortion.
2. Pre-eclampsia.
3. Preterm labour.
4. Discordant fetal growth.
5. Polyhydramnios.
6. Fetal anomaly.
7. Intra-uterine death.

Intrapartum factors associated with a twin pregnancy include an increased risk of:

1. Asphyxia.
2. Malpresentation of one or both twins.
3. Intra-uterine manipulation.
4. Instrumental delivery.
5. Caesarean section.
6. Postpartum haemorrhage.

18.2 MODE OF DELIVERY

The decision as to mode of delivery will depend upon many factors, including:

1. Previous obstetric history.
2. Maternal age.
3. Present pregnancy complications such as:
   a. IUGR.
   b. Pre-eclampsia.
4. Fetal presentations.
5. Maternal wishes.

The decision as to mode of delivery should be discussed fully with the patient and her partner antenatally. If vaginal delivery is considered appropriate, an outline of what the woman may expect in labour and advice as to suitable analgesia should be given before labour. The woman should be advised to attend hospital immediately she suspects she is in labour, particularly if she is multiparous.

18.3 MANAGEMENT OF LABOUR

During labour, the second twin is at particular risk because of its inaccessibility. It should be possible to monitor its heart rate as described below, but it is obviously impossible to estimate scalp pH when there is a CTG abnormality.

18.3.1 Investigations

A woman with a twin pregnancy should have blood taken for haemoglobin estimation, cross-matching of two units of blood and an intravenous infusion of Hartmann's solution commenced as soon as she is in established labour.

18.3.2 Monitoring

It is essential to monitor both fetal hearts during labour. It is not usually possible to achieve this with two external transducers, because the ultrasound beams interfere with each other. Therefore in early labour each twin should be monitored intermittently and alternately. As soon as it is safe to do so, the membranes of the leading twin should be ruptured, and a fetal scalp electrode applied. Both twins can then be monitored continuously, either with separate machines, or by a single machine especially suited for that purpose. In either case, it is important to establish that two differing heart rates are being recorded.

Continuous monitoring should occur until the time of delivery. If serious heart rate abnormalities of the second twin are observed, Caesarean section will be necessary.

18.3.3 Analgesia

Epidural block is the preferred analgesia for twin labour because:

1. It provides excellent analgesia and therefore good maternal co-operation. This is particularly important if intra-uterine manipulation of the second twin is necessary.
2. Instrumental assistance is likely to be necessary for one or both twins.
3. If a Caesarean section becomes necessary for reasons other than fetal distress the woman may have the option of epidural anaesthesia.

18.3.4 Augmentation

The same criteria for augmentation with syntocinon are used as for a singleton labour (see Chapter 8).

18.4 PREPARATION FOR DELIVERY

As the second stage approaches, an additional infusion of five units of syntocinon in 1000 ml Hartmann's solution is prepared and attached to the existing intravenous cannula by means of a three-way tap, which is *turned off*. The infusion pump is set to deliver the syntocinon at 20 drops min^{-1} but is turned off.

As the presenting part becomes visible, and/or the patient wishes to push, she should be prepared by being put into the lithotomy position with a 10° wedge under her left buttock. She should then be cleansed, draped with sterile towels, and the bladder emptied with a disposable catheter. Paediatric assistance is summoned in advance, *two* paediatricians being called to the delivery. The labour ward anaesthetist should also be present, but can wait outside the delivery room.

18.5 DELIVERY

The delivery should be attended by an obstetric registrar. The operator wears two pairs of surgical gloves for the delivery and the first twin is delivered in the usual manner after an episiotomy is performed. Syntometrine is *not* given. After clamping and dividing the cord and handing over the first twin, the operator palpates the maternal abdomen to determine the lie and presentation of the second twin. This may be confirmed by the use of the portable scanner if there is doubt.

18.5.1   Management of the second twin

18.5.1.1   IF THE LIE IS LONGITUDINAL

The operator removes one pair of gloves and performs a vaginal examination to confirm the abdominal findings. Either a foot, buttock or a head should be palpated. A second assistant should place their hands on either side of the patient's abdomen to stabilize the lie and slightly downward pressure will encourage the presenting part to enter the pelvis.

The syntocinon infusion should then be commenced if, as frequently happens, contractions have subsided. In the presence of efficient contractions, ARM is performed and the presenting part will descend into the pelvis. A fetal scalp electrode should be attached to the scalp, or a foot or buttock if the presentation is breech. Maternal pushing should then be recommenced.

As a general guideline the second twin should be delivered within 30 min of the first. Delay beyond this time leads to an increased incidence of intrapartum asphyxia and increases the possibility of the cervix clamping down onto the fetal head. Undue delay in delivery should therefore lead to a forceps delivery if the presentation is cephalic or traction on the feet or groins if the fetus is presenting by the breech. This is acceptable in the case of the second twin as the birth canal is already dilated by the passage of the first twin.

After delivery of the second twin the cord is clamped with different instruments so that the cords can be identified when the placenta and cords are examined.

18.5.1.2   IF THE LIE IS TRANSVERSE

External version should be attempted by an assistant who exerts firm pressure on the maternal abdomen to encourage the lie to become longitudinal. If this fails, the operator removes one pair of gloves, performs a vaginal examination, being very careful not to rupture the membranes, and attempts a combined internal and external version. If this fails he/she should grasp a foot through the membranes. A foot can be differentiated from a hand by feeling the heel. By grasping the foot and then performing ARM, internal podalic version and a breech extraction can be performed.

If the membranes rupture whilst the second twin lies transversely, internal version may be difficult and traumatic. If this occurs or if the fetus is presenting with its back down it may not be possible to perform an internal version so a Caesarean section will be necessary.

18.5.2   The immediate puerperium

After delivery of the second twin syntometrine is given and prophylaxis against a PPH as described in Chapter 13.

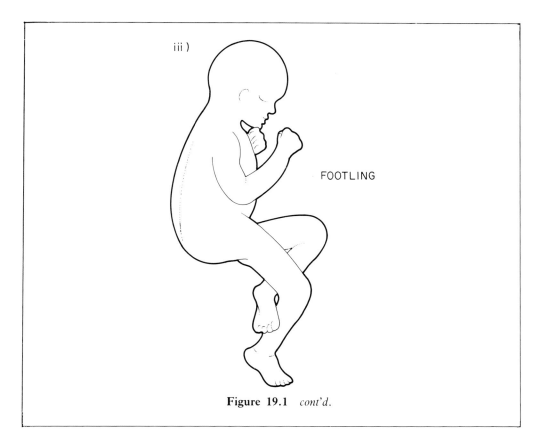

iii)

FOOTLING

Figure 19.1 *cont'd.*

been discussed antenatally as its use allows a more controlled delivery of the after-coming head. It is best to forewarn the patient that at any stage of the labour it may become necessary to perform a Caesarean section.

2. Perform an abdominal palpation to determine the presenting part and if it is engaged (i.e. the bitrochanteric diameter is below the pelvic brim).

3. Perform a vaginal examination to determine the cervical dilatation and confirm the presentation. *Do not rupture the membranes* until the presenting part is well down in the pelvis and the cervix is at least 4 cm dilated. This reduces the risk of cord prolapse. When recording the findings at vaginal examination in a breech presentation remember that the position is described with reference to the orientation of the fetal sacrum.

4. CTG monitoring should be continuous throughout labour.

5. Start an intravenous infusion of normal saline and send blood for:
   a.   Haemoglobin estimation.
   b.   Group and save serum.

6. Give the patient 150 mg ranitidine orally (with a small sip of water) every 6 h.

7. If the patient has agreed to epidural analgesia arrange for it to be performed.

8. Repeat the vaginal examination every 4 h. Rupture the membranes if the presenting part is deeply engaged and the cervix is more than 4 cm dilated. Attach a fetal scalp clip to the skin over the sacrum, or to the sole of a foot in the case of a flexed breech.

9. If the cervical progress in labour falls two hours or more to the right of Studd's nomogram perform a Caesarean section.
10. If the CTG is abnormal a fetal blood sample may be obtained from the breech and interpreted in the usual way (see Section 15.5.2).
11. Length of the second stage. If the patient has an effective epidural she may be allowed an hour in the second stage before she starts to push. Pushing should probably be limited to 45 min in a primipara and 30 min in a multipara. If delivery is not imminent after this time a Caesarean section should be performed.
12. Do not start the patient pushing until the breech is visible at the vaginal introitus.

19.4 MANAGEMENT OF A BREECH DELIVERY

1. If the patient has epidural analgesia ensure that it is topped up before delivery is imminent. If not, the minimum analgesia necessary is a pudendal block with local perineal infiltration.
2. Put the patient in the lithotomy position with a wedge under her left buttock to prevent the supine hypotension syndrome.
3. Summon the paediatrician and the anaesthetist.
4. Scrub up and put on sterile gloves. Open a delivery pack, cleanse, drape and catheterize the patient. Open a pair of midcavity forceps in readiness, e.g. Neville–Barnes forceps.
5. Ask the patient to start pushing and when the buttocks are distending the perineum cut a right medio-lateral episiotomy.

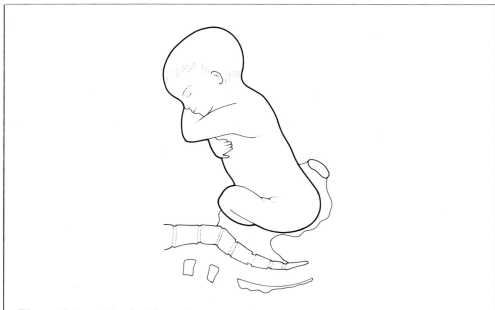

Figure 19.2   The fetal buttocks engaged in the oblique or transverse diameter of the pelvic brim

6. The mechanism of a normal vaginal breech delivery is illustrated in Figures 19.2 to 19.9. Allow the trunk to be delivered by uterine contractions and maternal effort to the point where the umbilical cord is visible. The sacrum will rotate anteriorly. Pull down a loop of cord to avoid undue traction on the cord at the umbilicus.

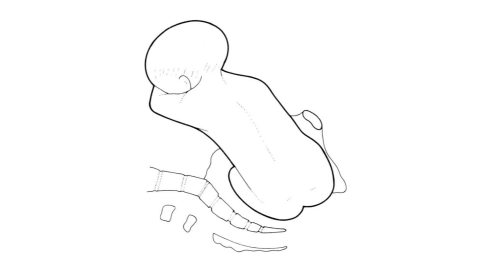

Figure 19.3   Internal rotation of the fetal buttocks on the pelvic floor has now occurred and the bitrocanteric diameter is now in the antero-posterior diameter of the pelvic outlet

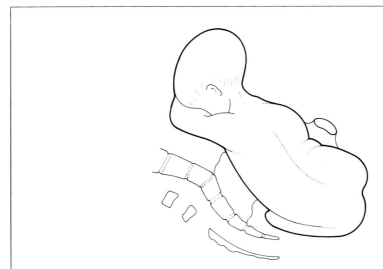

Figure 19.4   The anterior buttock appears at the vulva by lateral flexion of the fetal trunk around the maternal symphysis pubis. At this stage the posterior buttock distends the perineum and an episiotomy should be cut

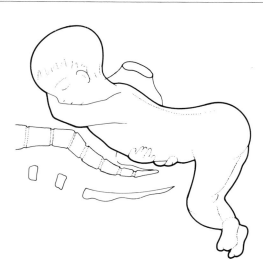

Figure 19.5   The buttocks are born and external rotation occurs as the shoulders engage in the transverse diameter of the pelvis

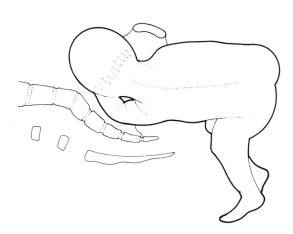

Figure 19.6   The shoulders rotate internally such that the bisachromial diameter lies in the anterio-posterior diameter of the outlet. The buttocks restitute by means of anterior rotation and then the head engages with the sagittal suture in the transverse diameter of the pelvic brim

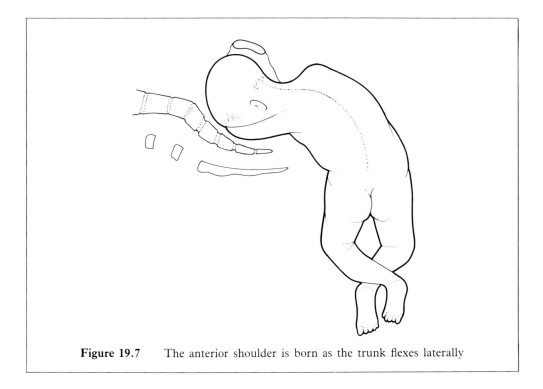

Figure 19.7   The anterior shoulder is born as the trunk flexes laterally

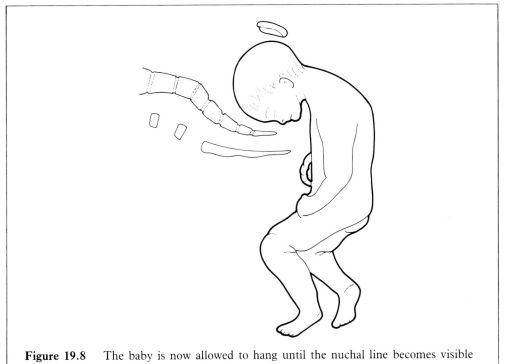

Figure 19.8   The baby is now allowed to hang until the nuchal line becomes visible

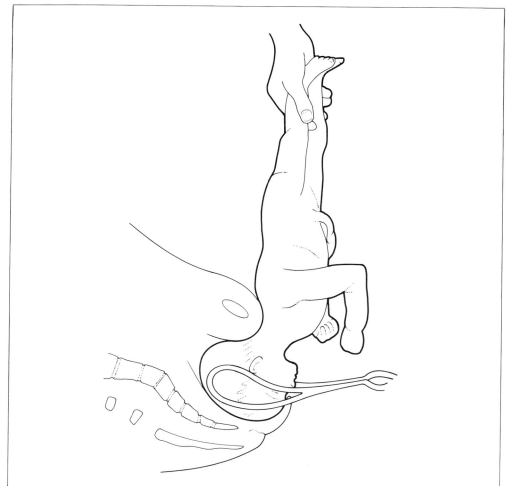

Figure 19.9   Prague's manoeuvre is performed by grasping the fetal ankles and sweeping them up towards the maternal abdomen. Midcavity forceps are then applied to the fetal head which is finally delivered by slight downward traction with flexion

7. Deliver the legs by splinting the femur between your index and middle finger and pressing behind the fetal knee. This will cause the knee to flex and the leg will deliver. *Never hook a fetal limb* as you will break the long bones.
8. Allow the remainder of the trunk to deliver up to the point where the shoulder blades are visible. The arms will usually be born spontaneously. If, however, the arms are extended they will be delivered by Lövset's manoeuvre: using a sterile towel, grasp the baby by placing your index and middle fingers on its anterior, superior iliac spines and your thumbs along the sacro-iliac joints. Using these points only rotate the baby through 180° such that the posterior shoulder now becomes anterior and escapes beneath the symphysis pubis. Pass your index and middle finger over the baby's shoulder, splint the humerus and deliver the arms

by gentle pressure in the baby's antecubital fossa. Rotate the infant back through 180° and deliver the other arm in the same manner.

9. Allow the infant to hang such that its own weight causes the head to enter the pelvis and the neck to flex (Figure 19.8). When the nuchal line (hair line) becomes visible grasp the baby's ankles between your thumb and middle finger with your index finger between the baby's legs and with gentle downward traction sweep the legs up in an arc over the maternal abdomen and hand the legs to an assistant. This manoeuvre (Prague's manoeuvre) will deliver the baby's mouth at the perineum and it should be aspirated with a mucus extractor by an assistant. *Note*: Do not be tempted to perform the Prague manoeuvre before the hair line is visible or the infant's mouth will not clear the perineum as the head will not have descended through the pelvis.

10. Apply forceps to the aftercoming head. They should be applied with the blades horizontal to the ground and not starting parallel with the inguinal ligament. Exert gentle downward traction and flex the fetal head to complete the delivery. The forceps should be used to achieve a slow controlled delivery of the infant's head.

19.5   UNDIAGNOSED BREECH PRESENTATION

Unless labour is advanced patients with a breech presentation that is diagnosed for the first time in labour should undergo an emergency erect lateral pelvimetry and an ultrasound examination to estimate fetal weight and to exclude major abnormalities.

If these facilities are not available an individual decision should be made. If the patient is a multipara who has delivered good sized babies (more than 3 kg) before she should be allowed an attempt at vaginal breech delivery. If, however, there is any doubt Caesarean section is the safest course.

19.6   FETAL RISKS OF BREECH DELIVERY

1. Intracranial haemorrhage from rupture of the falx cerebri or tentorium cerebelli due to a poorly controlled delivery of the fetal head.
2. Fracture of the clavicle, humerus or femur due to incorrect handling of fetal long bones.
3. Erb–Duchenne palsies due to traction on the arms before delivering them.
4. Ruptured abdominal viscus from incorrect handling.
5. Dislocation of the hip.

Chapter 20

Face, Brow, Shoulder and Compound Presentation

20.1 FACE PRESENTATION

20.1.1 Introduction

Face presentation is described as primary or secondary. A primary face presentation presents before the onset of labour, and the more common secondary face presentation develops during labour. With the modern tendency towards smaller families face presentation is now only seen in about one in 3000 deliveries.

20.1.2   Causes

1. The most common cause is probably a lax uterus leading to poor flexion of the fetal head. If this is associated with an occipito-posterior vertex presentation and there is also a dextrorotated uterus this tends to promote extension of the fetal head.
2. Fetal thyroid goitre.
3. Intra-uterine fetal death.
4. Multiple pregnancy.
5. Prematurity.
6. As a development from a brow presentation.
7. Anencephaly.

20.1.3   Mechanism

1. The engaging diameter of the face presentation is the submento-bregmatic (see Figures 20.1 and 20.2). The submento-bregmatic diameter is usually 9.5 cm which is the same as the suboccipito-bregmatic diameter of a fully flexed vertex presentation. The fetal face, however, will not mould in the same way that the vertex will so disproportion is more common.

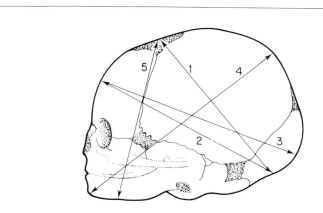

Diameter	Length	Presentation
1. Sub-occipito–bregmatic	9.5 cm	Flexed vertex
2. Sub-occipito–frontal	10.5 cm	Partially-deflexed vertex
3. Occipito–frontal	11.5 cm	Deflexed vertex
4. Mento–vertical	13.0 cm	Brow
5. Submento–bregmatic	9.5 cm	Face

Figure 20.1   Diameters of the fetal skull

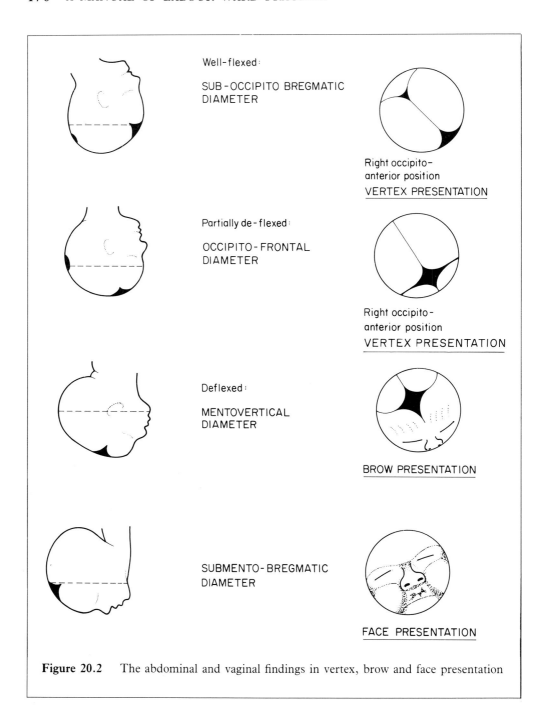

Figure 20.2 The abdominal and vaginal findings in vertex, brow and face presentation

2. Unless the chin rotates anteriorly (mento-anterior) the fetus will not deliver as the chin will impact in the sacral hollow, see Figure 20.3. This only applies to term fetuses and preterm fetuses may deliver from a mento-posterior position.
3. The face usually engages in the transverse diameter of the pelvic brim in a left

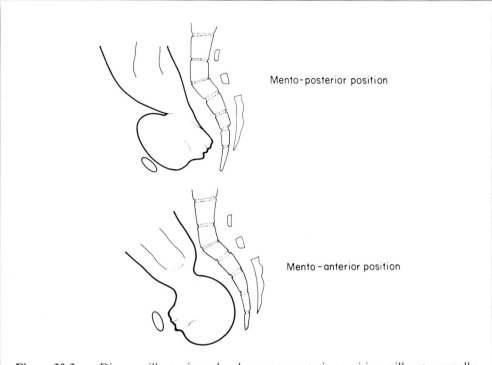

Figure 20.3   Diagram illustrating why the mento-posterior position will not normally deliver vaginally. The fetal chin impacts in the sacral hollow

mento-transverse (LMT) position. With increasing uterine action descent continues until the pelvic floor is reached where rotation occurs. Most commonly the mentum leads and rotates forwards (internal rotation) to the left mento-anterior position (LMA).

4. With further descent the rotation brings the mentum directly beneath the symphysis pubis. The chin then escapes under the pubis and pregressive flexion allows delivery of the head.
5. If the sinciput leads during engagement the mentum will rotate posteriorly into the hollow of the sacrum and labour will become obstructed.

20.1.4   Diagnosis

1. On abdominal palpation (see Figure 20.4) there is much more occiput than sinciput palpable in the lower pole of the uterus. In addition if the membranes have ruptured there is usually a prominent grove between the head and the fetal back.
2. On vaginal examination (see Figure 20.2) the face presentation is usually easily diagnosed. The hard fetal subra-orbital ridges are readily palpable and a finger can usually be inserted into the fetal mouth which is differentiated from the anus by the hard areolar ridges (the fetal gums). *Note*: Having diagnosed a face presentation further vaginal examinations should be performed without the use of Hibitane cream as this irritates the fetal eyes and may cause conjunctivitis.

20.1.5 Management of labour

1. Ideally all fetuses presenting by the face should have an ultrasound scan to exclude coexisting structural abnormalities.
2. The face is an ill-fitting presenting part so contractions in early labour are often infrequent. If the diagnosis is made at this stage the membranes should be left intact because of the risk of a prolapsed cord. Labour should be stimulated when progress falls more than 2 h to the right of the line of expected cervical dilatation (see Section 7.3).
2. The fetal heart should be continuously monitored and this is initially performed externally. At 5 cm or more of cervical dilatation ARM is performed and a fetal scalp electrode may be applied to the fetal forehead either by palpation or under direct vision by use of an amnioscope and a spiral electrode. Likewise if fetal blood sampling is necessary the sample should be taken from the fetal forehead.
3. Vaginal examination should be performed three hourly. Caesarean section is indicated for fetal distress or secondary arrest of cervical dilatation following adequate stimulation by syntocinon (see Section 7.3).
4. During the course of labour the face presentation may flex through a brow presentation to a vertex presentation.
5. If the mentum rotates posteriorly and there is abnormal progress despite syntocinon a Caesarean section should be performed. If the cervix reaches full dilatation and the face is low in the pelvis with a mento-posterior presentation it may be rotated manually or by the use of Kjelland's forceps.

20.2 BROW PRESENTATION

20.2.1 Introduction

Brow presentations are rare and probably now only occur about one in 5000 deliveries. This presentation is usually transient and will tend to convert to a face or a fully flexed vertex presentation by extension or flexion of the fetal neck respectively. The causes are similar to that of a face presentation.

Unless the pelvis is roomy or the baby is small, brow presentations rarely deliver vaginally because the presenting diameter (mento-vertical) is 13 cm (see Figures 20.1 and 20.2). If a brow presentation is diagnosed early in labour, labour should be allowed to progress and stimulated with syntocinon according to the usual criteria (see Section 7.3) as conversion to a face or vertex presentation may occur. If a brow presentation is diagnosed at full dilatation with a term baby the safest method of delivery is Caesarean section.

20.2.2 Diagnosis

1. On abdominal palpation (Figure 20.5) the head usually feels unduly large. On more detailed palpation the sinciput is not palpable.
2. On vaginal examination (Figure 20.2) the head is commonly high and the anterior fontanelle is usually encountered immediately beneath the examining fingers. The diagnosis of brow presentation is made by palpation of the supra-orbital ridges and the bridge of the nose.

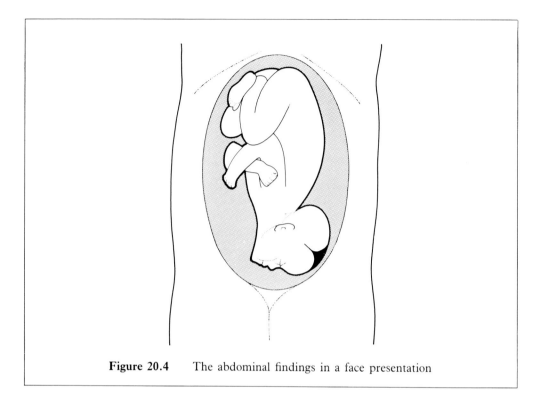

Figure 20.4   The abdominal findings in a face presentation

20.2.3 Management of labour

1. The brow is ill-fitting in the maternal pelvis so it is not uncommon for membranes to rupture early in labour with the associated risk of a cord prolapse.
2. If the diagnosis is made in early labour the progress of labour should be followed by three hourly vaginal examinations. If labour falls more than 2 h to the right of the line of expected cervical dilatation (see Section 7.3) a syntocinon infusion should be commenced. A further vaginal examination should be carried out after 3 h of full dose syntocinon and if no progress has been made Caesarean section should be performed.
3. If the cervical dilatation progresses normally, either spontaneously or in response to syntocinon, labour should be allowed to continue. In some cases flexion to a vertex presentation or extension to a face presentation will occur allowing subsequent vaginal delivery.

20.3 SHOULDER PRESENTATION

20.3.1 Introduction

This malpresentation only occurs in about one in 3000 deliveries and is more common in multipara and preterm labour.

20.3.2   Causes

1. Multiple pregnancy.
2. Polyhydramnios.
3. Placenta praevia.
4. Contracted pelvis.
5. Hydrocephaly.
6. An abnormal shaped uterus, for example a subseptate uterus.

20.3.3   Diagnosis

1. Findings on abdominal palpation are illustrated in Figure 20.6. The fundal height is usually less than expected and the head is located in one flank.
2. In early labour a vaginal examination usually reveals an empty pelvis although a hand or elbow may be felt. It is also common to feel the tip of the shoulder, the ribs or the greater trochanter of the fetus (see Figure 20.6).

20.3.4   Management

1. Any patient with a shoulder presentation should have an ultrasound examination to exclude placenta praevia and to ensure as far as possible that the fetus is structurally normal.
2. If the patient presents in early labour with intact membranes it may be possible to perform an external cephalic version. If this succeeds the fetus should be held

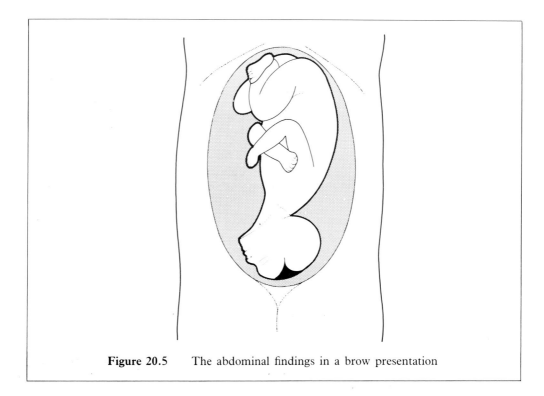

Figure 20.5   The abdominal findings in a brow presentation

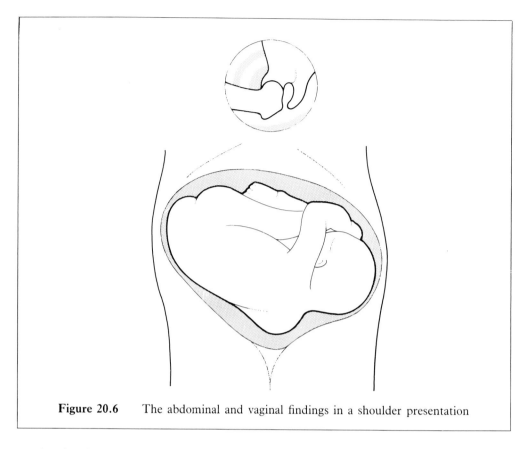

Figure 20.6   The abdominal and vaginal findings in a shoulder presentation

longitudinally and during the next contraction the membranes should be ruptured such that the head engages into the pelvis.
3.   If the membranes have ruptured or if labour is advanced then delivery is by Caesarean section.
4.   If the baby is dead, delivery should be by Caesarean section.

20.4   COMPOUND PRESENTATION

A compound presentation occurs when two or more parts of the fetus present. The most common are:

1.   A cephalic presentation with a hand or a foot.
2.   A breech presentation with a hand.

In both of the above cases the limb is usually held back at the pelvic brim as the presenting part descends.

More complex compound presentations are usually the result of a transverse or oblique lie. In early labour with intact membranes external cephalic version may be attempted otherwise delivery is by Caesarean section.

Chapter 21
Cord Prolapse

21.1 INTRODUCTION

Cord prolapse is an obstetric emergency. However, if dealt with promptly and appropriately in a properly-equipped labour ward, it should carry little added risk for the fetus.

21.1.1 Definitions

A *cord presentation* occurs when the umbilical cord presents below the presenting part of the fetus in the presence of intact membranes.

A *cord prolapse* occurs when the umbilical cord presents below the fetus in the presence of ruptured membranes. It may be palpable in the vagina, or in extreme cases it may be visible at the vulva.

21.2 PREVENTION OF CORD PROLAPSE

Most cases of cord prolapse are preventable by appropriate labour ward management. The situations in which this complication is more likely include:

1. At artificial rupture of membranes with a high presenting part.
2. In preterm labour (particularly with breech presentation).

3. With a breech presentation at any gestation (especially a footling breech).
4. With an unstable or transverse lie.

Therefore, in the management of normal labour rupture of the membranes should only be performed when the cervix is at least 4 cm dilated and the presenting part is engaged in the pelvis. All women should have a vaginal examination at the time of spontaneous rupture of the membranes to exclude a cord prolapse. Mode of delivery for the very low birth weight fetus presenting by the breech is controversial but many obstetricians will perform an elective Caesarean section thereby avoiding this complication (see Section 9.9).

Women who have a fetus with an unstable or transverse lie should be admitted to hospital from about 37 weeks' gestation, since spontaneous version to a cephalic presentation is unlikely after this time and the risk of spontaneous labour is high. If spontaneous rupture of the membranes should occur the patient should be examined to exclude a cord prolapse.

21.3   MANAGEMENT OF CORD PROLAPSE

21.3.1   Cord still pulsating

1. The person who detects the presence of a cord on vaginal examination should leave their hand in the vagina and elevate the presenting part, attempting to keep the cord within the uterus right up to the moment of delivery. This avoids compression of the cord and spasm of cord vessels caused by a drop in temperature, both of which cause fetal hypoxia. Whilst this is being done further assistance is summoned, and senior obstetric and anaesthetic staff are called to the labour ward.
2. The patient is put into an exaggerated left lateral position by a second person, with a pillow placed under the left buttock to raise the pelvis and prevent compression of the cord against the bony pelvis. Alternatively the knee–chest position may be used.
3. Arrangements are made for immediate delivery. If the cervix is fully dilated and the fetal head is well down a forceps delivery may be possible. If this is not the case, then Caesarean section is indicated. In a well-equipped and efficient labour ward delivery should be possible within 15 to 20 min.
4. An assistant should start an intravenous infusion of Hartmann's solution after taking blood for haemoglobin estimation and cross-matching of two units.

Cord prolapse is a situation when prompt action is essential. The presence of a cord presentation or prolapse is usually simple to diagnose, since the cord is characteristic and can be felt to pulsate if the fetus is alive. If the person who performs the original vaginal examination is doubtful about the diagnosis, then they should leave their hand within the vagina until a more senior person can take over and confirm the diagnosis.

It is important to remain calm under this situation and provide the patient with a brief explanation of what is happening without transmitting a feeling of panic. The staff involved with the case should make a point of returning to the patient after the delivery and spending time explaining why the complication had occurred and why that particular course of action was necessary.

21.3.2   No cord pulsation

If the cord prolapse occurred sometime before its detection, and particularly if the cord has prolapsed out of the vagina, the fetus may have died. The cord will no longer pulsate, and the diagnosis of intra-uterine death can be confirmed by real-time ultrasound scanning if possible.

1. Longitudinal lie, in established labour. Await full dilatation and descent in the second stage. Augment labour (see Section 7.3.3) if necessary, and provide adequate analgesia. An operative delivery performed when the presenting part is low in the pelvis is appropriate as it avoids maternal effort.
2. Longitudinal lie, not in established labour. Induce labour by means of a syntocinon infusion (see Section 7.3.3) and provide adequate analgesia.
3. Transverse or oblique lie. Unless skilled in destructive procedures deliver by Caesarean section. Attempts at internal or external version will fail because of the absence of amniotic fluid and risk uterine rupture.

21.4   MANAGEMENT OF CORD PRESENTATION

21.4.1   Cord alongside presenting part

Allow labour to progress as the descent of the presenting part will often push the cord out of the pelvis. If the membranes rupture perform an immediate vaginal examination to exclude a cord prolapse. *Note*: The fetal heart rate trace will often show variable decelerations (see Section 15.4.1) as a result of cord compression. In term infants this rarely results in asphyxia but may do in preterm infants so Caesarean section is advised.

21.4.2   Cord over or below presenting part

Deliver by Caesarean section.

Chapter 22

Uterine Inversion

22.1 INTRODUCTION

Uterine inversion is a very rare obstetric emergency, with an incidence of about one in 20 000 deliveries. It may be described by degrees (see Figure 22.1) or as incomplete or partial when the inverted uterus appears at the cervix, and complete when the whole uterus appears outside the vulva. The placenta is usually still attached, but may not be. It is a condition which results in profound shock and sometimes death and so must be dealt with promptly and efficiently.

22.2 ASSOCIATED FACTORS

1. Excessive cord traction during the third stage without guarding the uterus with countertraction over the suprapubic area with the opposite hand.
2. An abnormally adherent placenta (e.g. placenta accreta) particularly when it is implanted in the fundus.
3. Uterine atony.

Usually several of these factors contribute to the aetiology of an inverted uterus. Occasionally uterine inversion is said to occur spontaneously.

22.3 CLINICAL FEATURES

The patient is usually profoundly shocked but may complain of a severe deep aching pain in the lower abdomen, which is due to tension on the ovaries and pelvic peritoneum.

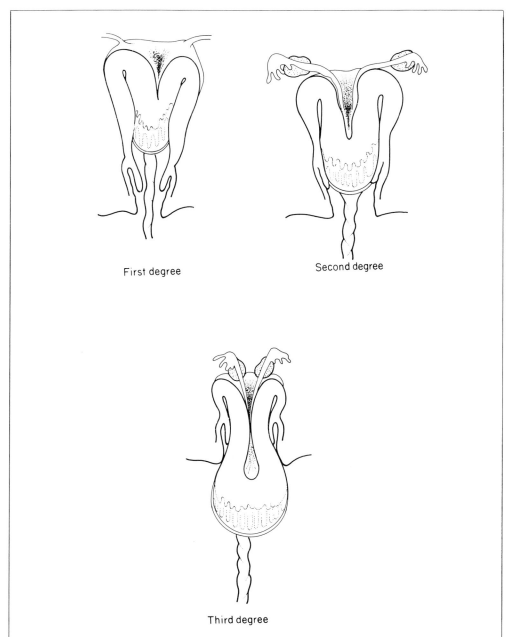

First degree

Second degree

Third degree

Figure 22.1   Acute inversion of the uterus. This may be classified in degrees as illustrated above or as partial (first and second degree) and complete (third degree)

There may be massive blood loss from the placental bed if the placenta has already been delivered.

22.3.1 Signs

The uterus will no longer be palpable per abdomen, and on vaginal examination the inverted fundus of the uterus is easily palpated.

22.4 MANAGEMENT

The following steps should be taken immediately:

1. Resuscitate the patient as described in Section 16.2.
2. If the placenta is already separated, the attendant should first attempt to replace the uterus within the vagina. This is done by exerting pressure on the fundus of the uterus with the palm of the hand in the direction of the long axis of the vagina.
3. If the placenta is still attached, it should not be removed until volume replacement has occurred. It is then manually separated from the uterine fundus after the uterus is replaced in the vagina as above.

If manual pressure will not replace the uterus in the vagina, a hydrostatic method can be used for partial inversion. A litre of sterile Hartmann's solution is connected to an ordinary giving set but the tubing is cut through close to the end, to remove the part which normally attaches to the intravenous cannula.

The tube is placed well into the vagina and the operator places both hands over the vulva, around the tube, forming a watertight seal (Figure 22.2). The sterile solution is run into the vagina as fast as possible and as hydrostatic pressure builds up, the uterus should be forced back into its correct position.

These measures may fail if:

1. The placenta is morbidly adherent.
2. There is a constriction ring of dense, oedematous tissue above the inverted uterus preventing its replacement.

In the first situation it may be possible to replace the uterus within the vagina, but attempted manual removal of the placenta would be unsuccessful. Bleeding will continue, and laparotomy is indicated. Hysterectomy may be the safest treatment.

When a constriction ring occurs, general anaesthesia is necessary. It may then be possible to replace the uterus with the relaxation produced by halothane anaesthesia. If not, laparotomy is necessary, and the constriction ring is carefully incised posteriorly to expose the fundus. A suture placed in the fundus may also be of assistance in exerting traction from above.

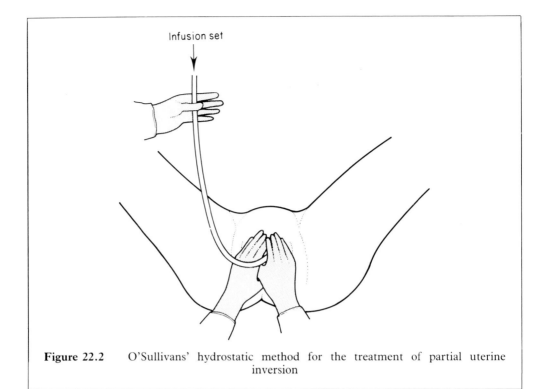

Figure 22.2   O'Sullivans' hydrostatic method for the treatment of partial uterine inversion

22.4.2   Subsequent management

1. After the uterus has been successfully replaced, measures to prevent further bleeding by ensuring a well-contracted uterus are taken as described in Chapter 13.
2. The bladder should not be allowed to become distended. An in-dwelling urethral catheter is therefore inserted and left for at least 24 h.
3. Bedrest for the first 24 h is advisable.
4. Prophylactic antibiotics, such as cephradine 250 mg q.d.s. and metronidazole 400 mg q.d.s. are also advisable.

Chapter 23
Uterine Rupture

23.1 INTRODUCTION

Uterine rupture is a serious obstetric complication with a high perinatal and maternal mortality. It is a largely preventable complication.

This complication is almost unheard of in primigravidae, but because some muscle is replaced by fibrous tissue in the multigravid uterus, these patients are more susceptible to rupture. This is particularly true if there has been previous uterine surgery and oxytocic drugs are used to induce labour or stimulate contractions.

The maternal mortality rate is 5 per cent, with a perinatal mortality rate at about 50 per cent.

23.2 CLASSIFICATION

1. Scar rupture, following:
   a. Caesarean section (either upper or lower segment).
   b. Hysterotomy.
   c. Myomectomy.
      Scars following myomectomy rarely rupture but are more likely to do so if the uterine cavity has been opened during the operation.
   d. Cornual resection of the fallopian tube for an interstitial ectopic pregnancy.
   e. Excision of uterine septum.
   f. Previous rupture repair.

2.   Traumatic rupture. This is usually the result of injudicious use of instruments or intra-uterine manipulation.
3.   Spontaneous rupture. This results from strong uterine contractions with or without oxytocic drugs, and with or without obstructed labour. These factors are often seen in combination.

The single most common associated factor in cases of uterine rupture is that of a previous Caesarean section scar. Rupture of the scar is more likely after a classical or upper segment incision, and less cmmon when the previous incision was in the lower segment, which is the non-contractile portion of the uterus. In the case of classical Caesarean section scars rupture may occur before the onset of labour.

If the rupture results in a laceration which communicates directly with the uterine cavity, the rupture is referred to as complete; if the visceral peritoneum is still intact over the uterine rupture, then it is termed incomplete.

23.3   PREVENTION

Prevention of uterine rupture depends upon the recognition of those circumstances under which the risk is significantly increased (see above). Obviously it will be impossible to prevent those unpredictable cases where rupture occurs before the onset of labour, but by modification of the management of labour, particularly with respect to oxytocic drugs, it may be possible to prevent rupture.

23.3.1   Scar rupture

Scar rupture during labour following hysterotomy or myomectomy is rare. In general an incision in a pregnant uterus has a greater risk of rupture during a subsequent labour than an incision made in a non-pregnant uterus. The risk following uterine perforation at the time of dilatation and curettage, for example, is negligible. The risk of scar rupture increases with an increasing number of previous Caesarean sections.

The presence or absence of peri-operative complications such as wound infection unfortunately provides no prediction about the strength of the Caesarean section scar. The extent of the uterus incision will contribute to subsequent risk of rupture; for example when difficulty is encountered during the delivery of the fetus at section and the incision in the uterus has to be extended to form a J- or T-shape this increases the risk of subsequent rupture, and elective Caesarean section is usually recommended for the next delivery. Likewise, elective Caesarean section is usually recommended following classical Caesarean section.

23.3.2   Traumatic rupture

Procedures associated with an increased risk of uterine rupture include:

1.   External cephalic version.
2.   Internal podalic version and breech extraction.
3.   Difficult forceps delivery (particularly rotational).

24.5   COMPLICATIONS OF SHOULDER DYSTOCIA

24.5.1   Fetal

1. Brachial plexus injuries, caused by excessive lateral flexion of the fetal neck.
2. Clavicular fractures, either accidental or deliberate.
3. Meconium aspiration.
4. Cord compression causing asphyxia.
5. Death.

24.5.2   Maternal

1. Cervical or vaginal lacerations.
2. Third degree tear.
3. Deliberate symphysiotomy, with subsequent urethral and bladder dysfunction.

Chapter 25
Maternal Injuries

25.1   INTRODUCTION

The following maternal injuries may be encountered after delivery:

1. Perineal and vulval tears. The recognition and repair of these is covered in Section 4.5. Third degree tears occur in about one in 200 deliveries.
2. Para-vaginal haematoma.
3. Rupture of the vaginal vault—colporrhexis.

4. Vaginal fistulae. Vesico-vaginal and recto-vaginal fistulae are extremely rare in developed countries. Their management is highly specialized and beyond the scope of this book.
5. Cervical tears.
6. Rupture of the uterus (see Chapter 23).
7. Acute inversion of the uterus (see Chapter 22).
8. Broad ligament haematoma.
9. Haematoma of the rectus sheath.
10. Traumatic neuritis—obstetric palsies.

25.2 THIRD DEGREE TEAR

This is a tear in which the whole anal sphincter is torn and is often accompanied by a tear of the rectal mucosa. If the injury is not recognized and repaired the patient will be incontinent of faeces.

It may occur either spontaneously or by extension of an episiotomy.

25.2.1 Management

1. Third degree tears are usually readily recognized if the rectal mucosa is also involved. If not the ends of the sphincter retract and the injury can be overlooked. If there is any doubt a finger inserted into the woman's rectum and gently pushed forward will reveal the absence of a sphincter.
2. Good analgesia is essential for an adequate repair. This means an effective epidural or a general anaesthetic.
3. The rectal wall is repaired with 2/0 chromic catgut on a round bodied needle (441). Interrupted sutures are used and are knotted inside the rectum (Figure 25.1).
4. The ends of the anal sphincter are then opposed with two or three No. 1 chromic catgut sutures.
5. The repair is then completed as for a second degree tear (see Section 4.6).

25.2.2 Postoperative management

It is now considered unnecessary to give laxatives or high residue diet.

If the repair breaks down, it should be left for at least six weeks before further repair is attempted.

The patient should have an elective episiotomy in the next pregnancy.

25.3 PARA-VAGINAL HAEMATOMA

Rupture of the veins of the vaginal plexus may produce a substantial haemorrhage into the para-vaginal space and extending downwards into the labium majorus. This may occur in the following circumstances:

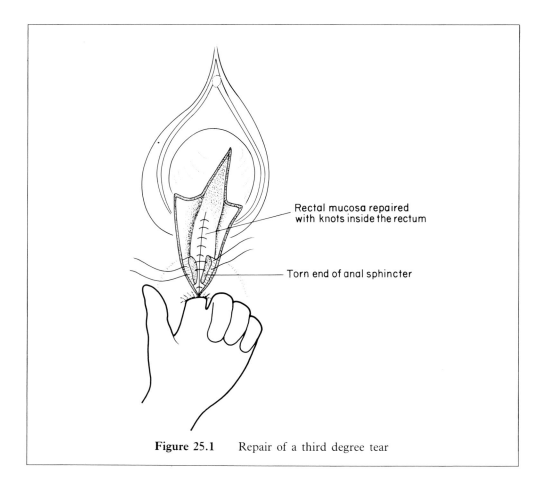

Figure 25.1   Repair of a third degree tear

1. After a precipitate delivery.
2. After instrumental delivery, particularly from the mid-cavity of the pelvis. The risk may be minimized if the delivery is controlled such that the vagina has time to dilate.
3. Following incorrect repair of an episiotomy. If the first stitch is not placed above the apex of the wound (see Section 4.4) a para-vaginal haematoma may result from a branch of the vaginal artery which has retracted above the wound.

25.3.1 Diagnosis

Para-vaginal haematomas may present as:

1. Collapse. The para-vaginal space may hold up to a litre of blood so the shock is out of all proportion to the visible blood loss.
2. Rectal pain, due to the haematoma pressing on the rectum.

The diagnosis is readily made as on vaginal examination the vaginal wall on the side of the haematoma is markedly deviated towards the midline and vaginal examination is very painful.

25.3.2 Management

1. If the patient is shocked treat the circulatory failure as described in Section 16.3.
2. Obtain good analgesia. This is usually by means of a general anaesthetic but as long as the patient has had adequate volume replacement an epidural (or spinal) anaesthetic may be used.
3. If the para-vaginal haematoma is on the side of the episiotomy take the episiotomy down. If not incise the vaginal wall over the entire length of the haematoma and evacuate the haematoma.
4. The individual bleeding point cannot usually be identified so the cavity should be repaired with interrupted No. 1 chromic catgut sutures. The vagina is then repaired with a continuous locked suture ensuring that the first suture is placed above the apex of the episiotomy or vaginal incision.
5. It is usually unnecessary to pack the vagina but if a pack is inserted the patient should be catheterized with a 14 or 16 FG Foley catheter with a 5–10 ml balloon. The pack and the catheter can be removed after 24 h.

25.4 COLPORRHEXIS—RUPTURE OF THE VAGINAL VAULT

This is usually due to incorrect application of the Kjelland's forceps such that the posterior blade perforates the posterior fornix of the vagina. It may also occur following obstructed labour in which case the tear is commonly in the lateral vaginal fornix.

25.4.1 Diagnosis

1. Most commonly the patient presents with either a postpartum haemorrhage or collapse with signs of intra-peritoneal haemorrhage.
2. If bleeding is not excessive it may be discovered at the time of examination under anaesthetic (EUA) for a postpartum haemorrhage. In this case the examining finger discovers the tear and then passes completely through it.

25.4.2 Management

1. Manage the circulatory collapse as described in Section 16.3.
2. Order at least six units of blood to be cross-matched.
3. Call a senior obstetrician who will then perform a laparotomy. If the bleeding points cannot be readily identified and ligated the uterine artery should be ligated at the level of the internal os. If this fails to control the bleeding ligate the internal iliac artery on that side. If bleeding is excessive or ligating the internal iliac artery fails a hysterectomy will be necessary.
4. If hysterectomy has not been necessary the vagina and, if necessary, the uterus should be repaired with interrupted No. 1 chromic catgut sutures.

5. If the patient has not had an in-dwelling catheter inserted before the laparotomy insert a 14–16 FG Foley catheter with a 5–10 ml balloon to measure urine output.

25.5 CERVICAL TEARS

The cervix is nearly always torn to some extent during delivery but these tears do not bleed and require no treatment. Severe cervical tears are associated with:

1. Instrumental delivery, especially if carried out before full cervical dilatation.
2. Previous cervical surgery which results in fibrous tissue which is more likely to tear.
3. A previous cervical tear.
4. Deliberate cervical incisions—now rarely performed but may be indicated if the cervix prevents the delivery of the after-coming head of a breech.

25.5.1 Diagnosis

This is suspected when a postpartum haemorrhage occurs in the presence of a well contracted uterus. The tear is usually discovered at examination under anaesthetic (EUA) as described in Section 13.4.1.

25.5.2 Repair

This is illustrated in Figure 25.2. The cervix is repaired with interrupted No 1 chromic catgut sutures.

25.6 BROAD LIGAMENT HAEMATOMA

This may occur in association with a ruptured uterus or with colporrhexis (rupture of the vaginal vault) in which case it is dealt with as part of the management of each condition.

Occasionally, a broad ligament haematoma will develop following rupture of the parametrial vessels at the time of vaginal delivery or because of inadequate haemostasis at the time of Caesarean section. In these cases the patient may present with:

1. Collapse due to blood loss into the broad ligament.
2. A high uterine fundus following delivery.

25.6.1 Diagnosis

This is made by the findings on abdominal palpation of:

1. A high uterine fundus that is deviated away from the side that contains the broad ligament haematoma.
2. An obvious mass arising from the pelvis and situated alongside the uterus.

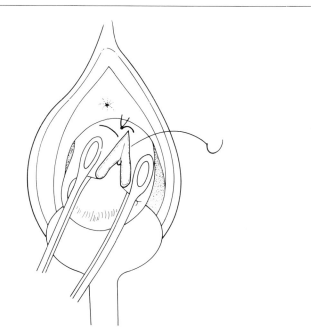

Figure 25.2   Repair of a cervical tear. The tear is demonstrated by grasping the cervix on either side between two pairs of sponge holding forceps. The tear is repaired with interrupted sutures of chromic catgut

25.6.2 Management

1. If the patient is shocked she should be resuscitated as described in Section 16.3.
2. If the patient has not had a visible postpartum haemorrhage it may safely be assumed that she has not sustained a rupture of the vaginal vault. Similarly, if the uterus is well contracted uterine rupture is unlikely.
3. The management is conservative as attempting to find the bleeding point at laparotomy is impossible and usually leads to hysterectomy. Having replaced the patient's circulating volume (see Section 16.3) she should be transfused with two units of fully cross-matched blood. In most patients there will be no further extension of the haematoma and it will gradually be resorbed over the course of four to six weeks.
4. Indications for surgical intervention are:
    a. Evidence of intra-peritoneal bleeding. This occurs soon after delivery. The patient will be shocked and the abdomen will be rigid with guarding and rebound tenderness.
    b. Extension of the haematoma which is suggested when transfusion does not keep the patient's vital signs stable.
    c. The subsequent development of a broad ligament abscess. This is very uncommon but the patient is obviously toxic with a high swinging pyrexia and

will have lower abdominal guarding and tenderness. If this occurs the broad ligament should be drained. The best approach is by opening the posterior wall of the inguinal canal and inserting a drain retro-peritoneally.

25.7   HAEMATOMA OF THE RECTUS SHEATH

This is a rare complication but occurs almost exclusively in multiparae as a result of strenuous pushing (or more commonly as a result of coughing or sneezing in the antenatal period). Muscle fibres and branches of the deep epigastric plexus are torn.

25.7.1   Diagnosis

The patient usually complains of pain following strenuous pushing. If the haematoma is above the umbilicus it is usually localized and readily palpable. If it is below the umbilicus, however, it may track anywhere along the transversalis fascia.

The blood loss may be sufficient to cause shock and in these cases the diagnosis is not usually made until a laparotomy is performed. Obvious blood clot will be located beneath the rectus sheath. The clot should be cleared out and the inferior epigastric vessels on that side should be ligated. The wound should be closed over a Redivac drain.

If the diagnosis is made without laparotomy the treatment is conservative; the haematoma being absorbed over four to six weeks. The diagnosis is readily confirmed by ultrasound examination (Figure 25.3).

25.8   TRAUMATIC NERVE PALSY

This is a rare condition in which one or both legs show evidence of motor and/or sensory nerve damage shortly after delivery. The lateral popliteal nerve (arising from L4 to S2) is most commonly affected.

25.8.1   Causes and management

1. Prolapse of an intervertebral disc. This is usually the disc sited between L4 and L5 or between L5 and S1. The patient usually complains of pain radiating down the back of their leg to the foot. Straight leg raising is usually limited to less than 90° and the ankle jerk is often diminished or absent. There will be sensory loss over the appropriate dermatomes (see Figure 3.3). The help of an orthopaedic or neurosurgeon should be sought.
2. Neuropraxia. This is a temporary nerve palsy resulting from prolonged compression of the nerve. It may be the result of pressure from the fetal head on the lumbosacral trunk, backward rotation of the sacrum during delivery causing stretching of the lumbosacral trunk or from forceful wandering of the posterior blade of Kjelland's forceps. In addition, it may occur if the popliteal nerve (which travels over the head of the fibula) is trapped against a lithotomy pole.

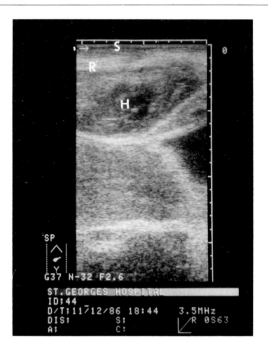

Figure 25.3   An ultrasound examination demonstrating a rectus sheath haematoma
(H = haematoma, S = skin)

In this case the patient will have foot drop and sensory impairment over the
relevant dermatomes (see Figure 3.3). Pain is not usually a prominent feature but
there may be tingling in the lower leg.

Recovery usually occurs within a few days and is aided by physiotherapy.

Chapter 26
Operative Delivery

26.1   INTRODUCTION

Operative delivery is the term for intervention during labour in the form of:

1. Instrumental delivery.
    a.   Ventouse extractor.
    b.   Forceps.
2. Caesarean section.
    a.   Emergency.
    b.   Elective.

There are many varieties of instruments available for delivery and it is important that the staff on the labour ward should be conversant with the instruments that they use. These are as follows:

1. Straight, mid cavity forceps such as Neville–Barnes, (Anderson's, Simpson's) (see Figures 26.1 and 26.2).
2. Outlet forceps such as Wrigley's (see Figure 26.3).
3. Kjelland's (see Figures 26.4 and 26.5).
4. Ventouse (vacuum) extractor (see Figure 26.6).

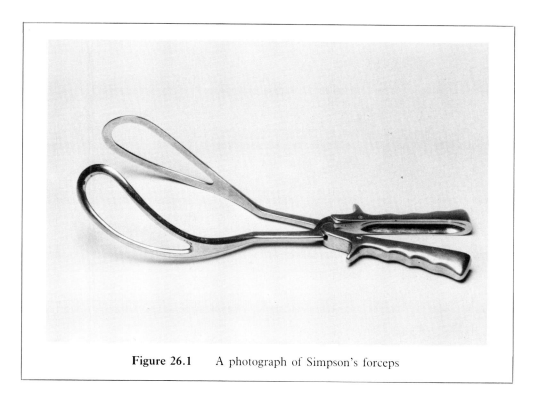

Figure 26.1   A photograph of Simpson's forceps

The indications for all operative deliveries are similar. Delivery before full dilatation is usually performed by Caesarean section (or very rarely by Ventouse extraction) and after full dilatation is performed by forceps or Ventouse. In general the choice between forceps or Ventouse depends upon the skill and preference of the operator.

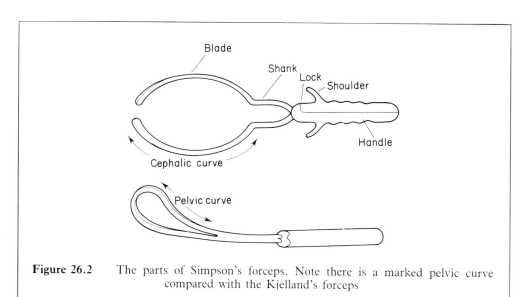

Figure 26.2   The parts of Simpson's forceps. Note there is a marked pelvic curve compared with the Kjelland's forceps

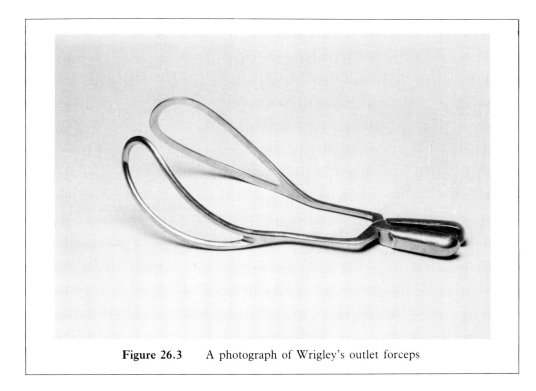

Figure 26.3   A photograph of Wrigley's outlet forceps

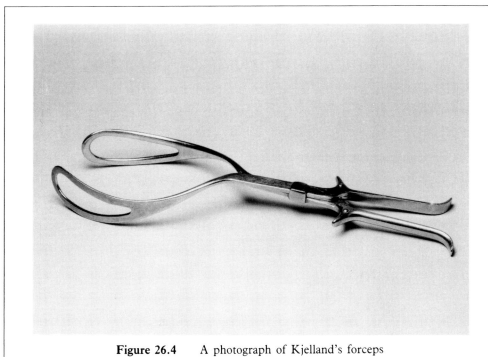

Figure 26.4   A photograph of Kjelland's forceps

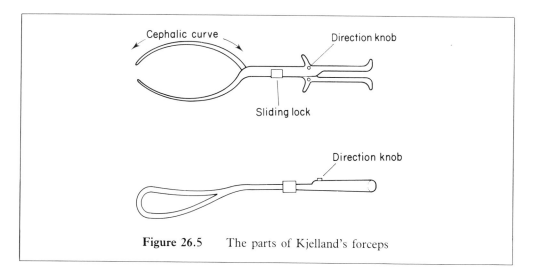

Figure 26.5   The parts of Kjelland's forceps

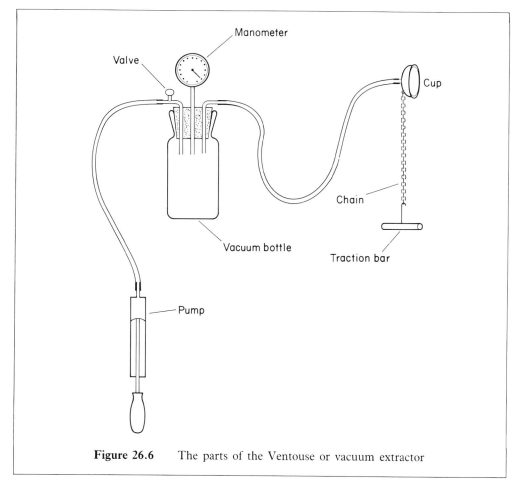

Figure 26.6   The parts of the Ventouse or vacuum extractor

26.2   INDICATIONS FOR OPERATIVE DELIVERY

1. Fetal distress. This is suspected by CTG abnormalities and whenever possible should be confirmed by means of a fetal scalp pH (see Sections 15.4 and 15.5).
2. Abnormalities of labour that fail to respond to syntocinon (see Section 8.2).
3. Maternal distress. This is a rare indication in well managed labours. It is defined as a rise in maternal temperature and pulse in the absence of infection. It is usually the result of dehydration (see also Section 8.1).
4. Maternal exhaustion. This is uncommon in the first stage of labour but may occasionally occur when adequate analgesia has not been obtained. In the second stage it usually results from allowing or encouraging the patient to push when the fetal head is still high within the pelvis (see Section 1.8).

26.3   CRITERIA FOR FORCEPS DELIVERY

1. No more than one-fifth of the fetal head should be palpable per abdomen (see Figure 1.1).
2. There should not be excessive moulding.
3. There should be adequate analgesia (see Table 26.1).
4. The person performing the delivery should have had adequate experience with that particular instrument or be supervised as deemed appropriate. This is particularly true for Kjelland's forceps.
5. The maternal bladder should be empty.
6. If the forceps is to result in delivery from the mid cavity there should be no evidence of fetal distress. Ideally prior to such delivery, especially if it is to be performed as a trial of forceps a fetal scalp pH should be obtained and if it is less than 7.2 delivery should preferably be by Caesarean section.

26.4   PROCEDURE FOR FORCEPS DELIVERY

1. Confirm that the above criteria for forceps delivery apply.
2. Explain the reason for intervention to the woman and her partner.
3. If the woman has an epidural block and the need for delivery is not urgent she

Table 26.1   Analgesia required for operative deliveries

Type of delivery	Minimum analgesia
1. Outlet forceps or Ventouse	Infiltration of the line of the proposed episiotomy and the posterior wall of the vagina
2. Mid cavity forceps or Ventouse	Pudendal block and infiltration of the line of the proposed episiotomy
3. Mid cavity rotational forceps	Epidural, caudal or spinal block or general anaesthesia
4. Breech delivery	Infiltration of the line of the proposed episiotomy

should be given a top-up in the sitting position in order to maximize perineal analgesia. It is usual to give 10 ml of 0.5 per cent plain bupivicaine (Marcain). This dose usually results in both sensory and motor blockage and therefore is ideal for forceps delivery.

4. Put the woman in the lithotomy position (see Figure 26.7) with a wedge under her right buttock in order to avoid the supine hypotension syndrome.
5. Clean the vulva with an antiseptic solution such as Savlon.
6. Place sterile drapes over the woman's legs and perineum.
7. Empty the bladder using a small disposable catheter with a sterile, no touch technique.
8. Perform a vaginal examination to confirm full dilatation, the position of the fetal head and the degree of moulding. Perform a bimanual examination to confirm that the head is fully engaged and that less than one-fifth is palpable in the abdomen.

   If the head is still palpable the procedure should be abandoned and delivery should be by Caesarean section (or possibly, by means of the Ventouse extractor).
9. Pudendal block and perineal infiltration should be performed if appropriate (see Table 26.1).
10. The appropriate instrument is selected and applied between contractions. The fetal head is rotated if necessary.
11. Traction should be applied with maternal effort during contractions. This is a general guideline but in situations of severe fetal distress traction should be applied

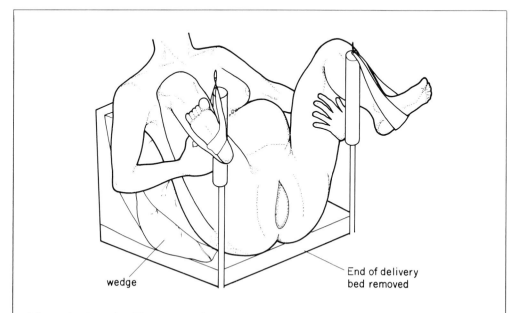

wedge

End of delivery
bed removed

Figure 26.7   An illustration of the lithotomy position used for forceps or Ventouse delivery. Note that the wedge placed under the woman's right buttock avoids the supine hypotension syndrome

immediately. Delivery should be accomplished over three to four contractions at most.

12. Once the fetal head distends the perineum an episiotomy should be performed.

13. After delivery of the head the instruments are removed and the body should be delivered in the usual way.

26.5 GUIDELINES ON THE APPLICATION OF INSTRUMENTS

26.5.1 Straight forceps

These instruments are used for non-rotational deliveries and possess both a cephalic and pelvic curve. Many operators prefer the Simpson's forceps for both mid and low cavity deliveries because the small handle and very shallow curve of the Wrigley's forceps may make it difficult to apply effective traction. The method of application of straight forceps is as follows:

1. The blades should be assembled in front of the patient but out of her direct line of vision. The left blade is selected and held in the operator's left hand with the handle parallel to the woman's right inguinal ligament. The operator's right hand is inserted into the vagina between the fetal head and the lateral wall (Figure 26.8a). The aim of this hand is to guide the blade into place and protect the vagina from damage. The blade should now be slid into position without the use of force. The right blade is then similarly applied and the instrument should lock together.

2. A vaginal examination should be performed to check that the blades lie equidistant from the sagittal suture. If there is any difficulty in application or if the blades do not lock then an undiagnosed malposition is likely. In this case the blades should be removed and a repeat vaginal examination should be performed to confirm the position.

3. If the fetal position is right occipito-anterior or left occipito-anterior straight forceps may still be used and are applied as indicated in Figures 26.9a and b. It is usually unnecessary to correct the rotation as traction will convert the position to direct OA as the head descends.

4. Figure 26.10 illustrates the way in which the hands should be applied to the forceps before traction is applied. The operator's left hand applies no traction but rests on the forceps in order to ensure that the direction of traction is in the line of the pelvic curve. Many operators prefer to use an underhand grip with the right hand as traction is then applied by use of triceps and this lessens the likelihood of applying excessive traction.

5. Traction is applied in the direction as indicated in Figure 26.11 until the head descends onto the perineum.

6. As the head descends onto the perineum the direction of traction is now slightly more upwards in order to encourage fetal head extension. All traction with forceps deliveries should be controlled and slow in order to give time for the vagina to adequately dilate and to avoid sudden decompression of the fetal head at delivery. As the fetal head distends the perineum the episiotomy should be cut and delivery is completed by further extension of the fetal head.

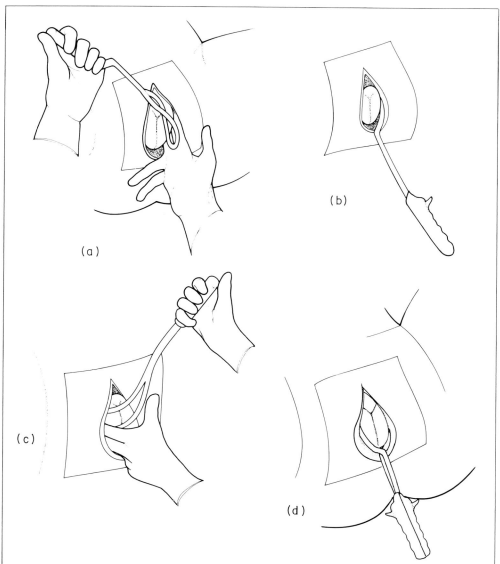

(a)

(b)

(c)

(d)

Figure 26.8   The method of application of the forceps for low or mid cavity
(a) The index and middle finger of the operator's right hand are inserted into the vagina between the fetal head and the lateral wall. The left blade of the forceps is then held parallel with the patient's inguinal ligament and guided into position.
(b) The left blade in position.
(c) The right blade being inserted in a similar manner.
(d) Both blades now in position and equidistance from the sagittal suture

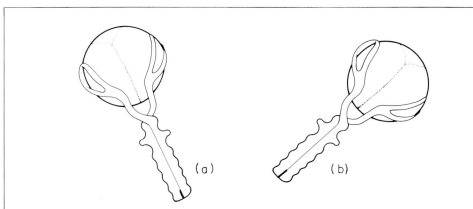

Figure 26.9   The method of applying the blades if the position of the head is not quite direct occipito-anterior.
(a) For a right occipito-anterior position.
(b) For a left occipito-anterior position

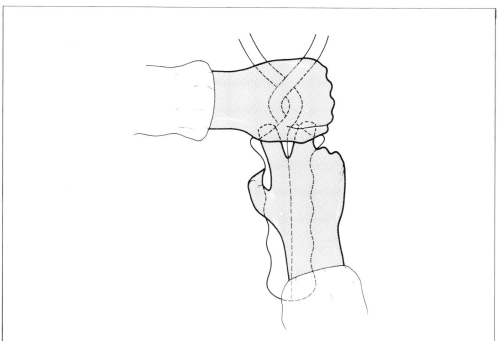

Figure 26.10   The method of applying the hands to the forceps such that traction can be exerted

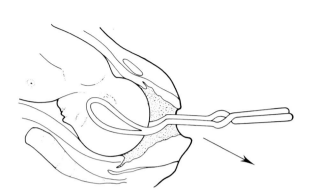

Figure 26.11   The direction of traction. This is the direction in which traction should be exerted if delivery is to be from mid cavity. As the head crowns the direction of traction should be such that extension of the fetal head is encouraged

26.5.2   Kjelland's forceps

These forceps are used for rotational delivery. They require good analgesia which must be an epidural, caudal or spinal block or a general anaesthetic. Pudendal block is not sufficient as rotation of the fetal head occurs in the mid-cavity, which is above the level at which the pudendal nerve is blocked. The lower extent of the mid cavity is indicated by the ischial spines and it is below this point that the pudendal nerve is blocked. Inadequate analgesia will lead to difficulty in applying the forceps and pain as rotation occurs because the fetal head crushes the sacral plexus.

1.   The Kjelland's forceps are assembled in front of the patient but out of her direct line of vision. The small metal knobs (see Figure 26.5) should be directed towards the occiput.
2.   Occipito-posterior position. In this case the blades are inserted as though they were straight forceps but with the direction knobs towards the fetal occiput. If the head is not quite directly occipito-posterior it should be marginally rotated such that this position is achieved. Traction should then be applied with contractions and if the head will easily deliver in the OP position this is preferable to rotating it. If no descent occurs then an attempt should be made to rotate the head. The choice of whether the head is rotated clockwise or anti-clockwise is usually determined by the position of the head. For example if the head was ROP then clockwise rotation should be attempted first. If rotation in one direction fails then it should be attempted in the other direction. If this fails the procedure should be abandoned, the fetal head should be pushed up into the pelvis and a Caesarean section should be performed.
3.   Occipito-transverse positions. The method of application of the Kjelland's forceps in this situation is as indicated below and in Figures 26.12(a)–(g).
    a.   Having determined the position of the fetal head and confirmed it by feeling a fetal ear the forceps should be assembled in front of the patient with the

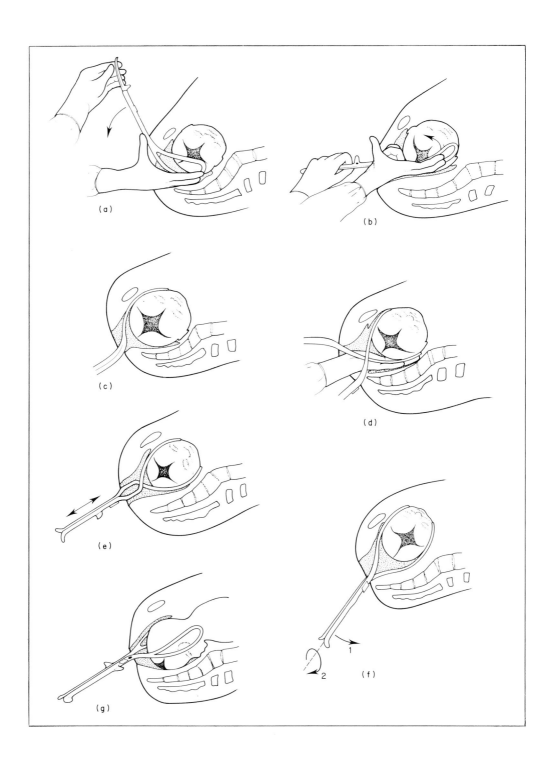

direction knobs pointed towards the occiput. The anterior blade is then selected and is applied over the baby's face as illustrated in Figure 26.12(a). If the position is ROT the blade is held in the operator's left hand whilst the right hand is inserted in the vagina in order to guide the blade and to protect the vaginal mucosa.

b.   The handle of the Kjelland's blade is then lowered as far as possible and using the middle and index finger of the hand which is in the patient's vagina the blade is wandered round until it comes to lie over the parietal eminence (Figures 26.12(b),(c)).

c.   The operator's right hand is then inserted into the vagina behind the baby's head and as far into the sacral hollow as possible. The posterior blade is then inserted and guided past the sacral promontory by means of the hand in the vagina. The blades are then locked and any asynclitism is corrected by sliding the blades until the handles are aligned (Figure 26.12(e)).

d.   A vaginal examination is performed to confirm that the blades are equidistant from the sagittal suture and are in appropriate positions. The handles are then depressed (Figure 26.12(f)) and using the finger and thumb of the right hand on the forceps handles an attempt is made to rotate the head in the shortest direction to achieve a DOA position.

e.   After the rotation is completed a vaginal examination should be performed to confirm that the posterior fontanelle is palpable and that the blades are still equidistant from the sagittal suture. Failure to feel the occipital fontanelle usually indicates that the forceps have rotated around the fetal head. They should be removed and re-applied. The direction knobs on the Kjelland's forceps should now be seen to be uppermost (Figure 26.12(g)). Traction is then applied with the blades as far down as possible.

f.   Some operators prefer to apply the posterior blade of the Kjelland's forceps first as it is not uncommon to knock the anterior blade out of position during its application.

g.   Although some advocate cutting an episiotomy in order to assist with the application of the blades or the rotation we do not. We feel that the episiotomy

Figure 26.12   The method of use of Kjelland's forceps.
(a) The anterior blade is selected and inserted as for a mid cavity forceps delivery.
(b) The handle of the forceps blade is now lowered and using the index and middle finger of the operator's right hand the blade is wandered so it comes to lie over the parietal eminence.
(c) When the blade is in the correct position the directional knob faces towards the fetal occiput.
(d) The posterior blade is now applied directly.
(e) The blades are now slid until the asyncylitism is corrected.
(f) The blades are now lowered (1) and then the rotation is performed (2).
(g) When the rotation is complete the directional knobs should be seen orientated towards the fetal occiput. Before traction is applied a vaginal examination should be performed to confirm that rotation has occurred and that the blades are equidistant from the sagittal suture.

should only be cut when the rotation is complete and the head has been pulled through the vagina such that it distends the perineum. If this guideline is followed then the situation of a failed Kjelland's forceps delivery resulting in a Caesarean section, so that the woman has both an abdominal and perineal wound, is avoided.

h. Failed rotation. If it is not possible to rotate the head in the shortest direction to DOA then an attempt should be made to rotate it through 270° to DOP. If this fails traction should be applied to the Kjelland's forceps such that the fetal head is brought lower into the pelvis. A further attempt should be made to rotate the head. If failure occurs at this stage it is wise to abandon the procedure and deliver the baby by Caesarean section (remembering to disimpact the fetal head from the pelvis before taking the woman to theatre). A few obstetricians will suggest attempting a rotation at a higher plane in the maternal pelvis. Unless you are experienced in this it is not wise as it is possible to dislodge the head completely from the pelvis, possibly resulting in a traumatic high forceps rotation and delivery, and a risk of cord prolapse.

i. Post delivery. Following rotational delivery using Kjelland's forceps the cervix and vagina should be inspected for tears as detailed in Section 25.5.

26.6   THE VENTOUSE EXTRACTOR

The indications and criteria for use of the vacuum extractor are exactly as for forceps delivery but in addition some obstetricians consider that it may be applied before full dilatation. We would not advise this for the following reasons:

1. If the need to deliver the baby before full dilatation is for fetal distress it is extremely dangerous to embark on a potentially difficult mid cavity delivery. Genuine fetal distress results in a high P_{CO_2} which causes distension of the cerebral veins. Applying the Ventouse in this situation may result in an intracranial haemorrhage.

2. For failure to progress. The concern in this case is that there is unrecognized cephalo-pelvic disproportion. Clinical pelvimetry and assessing the degree of moulding does not accurately warn even experienced obstetricians that there is disproportion. We would therefore suggest that you manage abnormal labour as detailed in Chapter 8 and that failure to respond to syntocinon should lead to Caesarean section.

For those who consider that they have sufficient skill to apply the Ventouse before full dilatation in spite of the above warnings then the following additional criteria to those required for a forceps delivery should apply:

1. There should be no more than two-fifths of the fetal head palpable.
2. The cervix should be 6 cm or more dilated and the biparietal diameter should have passed through the vaginal vault.

26.6.1   Method

The relevant parts of the Ventouse extractor are illustrated in Figure 26.6. The largest cup (usually the 5 cm cup) should be selected and should be inserted into the vagina such that it comes to lie with its centre over the occipital fontanelle. The cup is held over the occiput and its margins are carefully checked by digital examination to ensure that no vaginal folds or parts of the cervix are trapped beneath it.

Negative pressure is then induced by an assistant. The pump should be operated until the manometer reads 0.2 kg cm^{-2}. At this stage the operator should re-examine the cup to ensure that it fits well onto the fetal head and that there is no part of the cervix or vagina trapped. The assistant then increases the pressure to 0.8 kg cm^{-2} in 0.2 kg increments at 2 min intervals. After a further 2 min the traction can be applied as illustrated in Figure 26.13 timed to coincide with uterine contractions and maternal effort. The left hand of the operator steadies the cup and provides slight counter traction while the right hand exerts traction in the line of the pelvic axis. As the fetal head descends onto the perineum an episiotomy should be cut and then the line of traction is gradually brought more anterior to encourage flexion of the fetal head. After

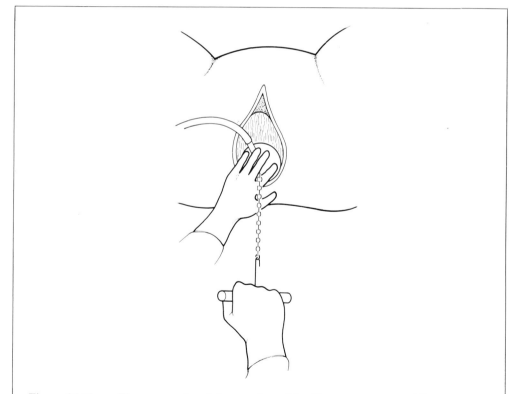

Figure 26.13   The means of applying traction with a Ventouse extractor. The operator's left hand steadies the cup whilst the right hand exerts traction in the line of the pelvic axis

delivery of the head the cap is removed by release of the vacuum and the body is delivered in the usual way.

It is important to warn the parents that the baby will have a chignon where the scalp was drawn up into the cup of the Ventouse. This usually disappears in the next 24 h.

26.7   INDICATIONS FOR INSTRUMENTAL DELIVERY IN OTHER CIRCUMSTANCES

Elective operative delivery is usually performed for the following reasons:

1. Following a dural tap. In this case maternal effort will increase the loss of cerebrospinal fluid and result in a severe headache.
2. Maternal hypertension. If the patient is hypertensive sufficient to require intravenous agents, bearing down efforts should be avoided as this increases the risk of a cerebrovascular accident. Elective forceps delivery should be performed when the fetal head has reached the outlet.
3. Maternal cardiac disease. If the mother has latent pulmonary oedema, suggested by crepitations at the lung base or evidence of frank pulmonary oedema then an elective outlet forceps delivery is preferable.
4. Proliferative retinopathy in a diabetic. Elective outlet forceps delivery is advised as maternal effort may rupture the fragile new vessels formed in the eye resulting in vitreous haemorrhage and possible blindness.
5. For the after-coming head in a breech delivery (see Section 19.4).
6. To assist in delivery of the head at Caesarean section.

26.8   INDICATIONS FOR CAESAREAN SECTION

Caesarean section is indicated for the following reasons:

1. When there is a need to avoid labour for maternal and/or fetal reasons.
   a. Placenta praevia. Major degrees of placenta praevia should result in Caesarean section because of the risk of severe bleeding (see Section 12.3.4).
   b. Previous Caesarean sections. Following two lower segment or one classical Caesarean section delivery should be by elective Caesarean section in the next pregnancy because of the risks of uterine rupture.
   c. Selected cases of breech presentation. Many obstetricians will electively deliver all breech presentations by Caesarean section. If, however, vaginal breech delivery is allowed in your unit then the contraindications are listed in Section 19.2.
   d. Severe intra-uterine growth retardation. Infants who have ceased growing completely antenatally are likely to get fetal distress in early labour and many obstetricians will opt for an elective Caesarean section.
   e. A successful operation for incontinence or prolapse. In this case it is preferable to deliver the patient by Caesarean section rather than to risk a recurrence of the incontinence or the prolapse.

f.   Transverse or oblique lie. In this case Caesarean section is preferred to attempting a stabilizing induction.
2.   To expedite delivery for fetal distress.
3.   In abnormal labour which has failed to respond to syntocinon (see Section 8.2).
4.   In the presence of an acute attack of genital herpes simplex. In this situation it is preferable to deliver the infant by Caesarean section to prevent it from acquiring systemic herpes during vaginal delivery. If the membranes have been ruptured for more than 4 h, however, the opportunity has been missed and Caesarean section will not avoid neonatal infection.

The method for performing a Caesarean section is outside the scope of this book and the reader is referred to textbooks of operative obstetrics.

II

COMPLICATED LABOUR

B. Maternal Disease

Chapter 27

Diabetes Mellitus

27.1   INTRODUCTION

Diabetes complicating pregnancy requires careful pre-pregnancy and antenatal preparation, the details of which are outside the scope of this book. The care of the patient must, however, extend to the labour ward as labour and delivery may result in metabolic upset.

Diabetes in pregnancy may be complicated by:

1. Fetal abnormality. Ideally, this should have been excluded as far as possible by detailed ultrasound examination in the first half of pregnancy. If not, major anomalies may be excluded by use of a portable real-time ultrasound machine when the patient presents in labour.
2. Polyhydramnios. This may lead to preterm labour, unstable lie, abnormal presentation, cord prolapse and postpartum haemorrhage.
3. Preterm labour. Preterm infants born to diabetic mothers are more likely to develop severe hyaline membrane disease and the management of preterm labour in diabetics is complicated by the fact that tocolytic agents and steroids are gluconeogenic.
4. Pre-eclampsia. This is not only more common in diabetics but tends to present earlier in pregnancy and to be more severe than in non-diabetic patients.
5. Macrosomia. This may be recognized antenatally by serial ultrasound examinations

or may be suspected from abdominal palpation. It may lead to shoulder dystocia (see Chapter 24) and birth trauma.

6. Sudden intra-uterine death. This may occur in the last four weeks of pregnancy but does not occur in well-controlled diabetics.
7. Neonatal problems:
   a. Hypoglycaemia.
   b. Hypocalcaemia.
   c. Hypothermia.
   d. Polycythaemia.
   e. Prematurity.
   f. Respiratory distress syndrome.
   g. Birth trauma.
   h. Congenital abnormalities.

27.2 MANAGEMENT OF LABOUR IN INSULIN-DEPENDENT DIABETICS

27.2.1 Spontaneous labour

1. All diabetics are high risk patients and so should have a constant labour attendant and continuous electronic fetal heart rate monitoring. They should also receive prophylaxis against Mendelson's syndrome as detailed in Section 3.8.
2. On admission the patient should be reviewed by the obstetric registrar. If the hospital has a combined antenatal clinic for diabetics it is usual practice to inform both the consultant obstetrician and consultant physician who run the clinic.
3. Obtain a capillary blood sample by finger prick and test it with a BM stick or a Dextrostix. Most diabetic patients will prefer to do this themselves. If a reflectance meter is available it should be used. It is unnecessary, however, to check the results by means of a venous sample sent to the laboratory.
4. Take venous blood for haemoglobin estimation and request that the serum is saved.
5. Start an intravenous infusion of normal saline and a second infusion made up as follows:
   a. 1 ℓ of 10 per cent dextrose.
   b. 30 units of soluble insulin.
   c. 2 g (26 mmol) potassium chloride (KCl).
   Note: The needles that are supplied with insulin syringes are not long enough to pierce the membrane of the drug portal of the infusion bag. Therefore draw up the insulin using a 1 ml syringe with a Luer lock and put into the infusion bag by means of a green needle through the drug portal.
   Run the infusion through an Ivac pump at 30 drops min^{-1} (90 ml h^{-1}).
6. Check the capillary blood sample using BM sticks or Dextrostix every 30 min. The aim is to keep the capillary glucose levels in the range 3–10 mmol ℓ^{-1}. In order to achieve this the solution should be altered based on Table 27.1.
   Note: Although this appears wasteful in that it may be necessary to discard partially-used infusion bags, it is safer to follow this practice if the insulin needs to be altered. If the infusion is accidentally turned off or disconnected the patient receives

Table 27.1   Control of diabetes in labour. Aim: capillary glucose levels of
3–10 mmol ℓ^{-1}

Glucose result (mmol ℓ^{-1})	Amount of soluble insulin (units) added to 1 ℓ 10 per cent dextrose with 2 g KCl
< 5	10
5–10	30
10–20	40
>20	50

nothing whereas if the insulin and dextrose are given through separate infusions accidentally discontinuing one solution may lead to coma.

7. Record the volume of all urine voided and test it for ketones and protein.

8. *Analgesia.* Epidural analgesia is recommended for all diabetics in labour for the following reasons:
   a. Pain causes catecholamine release which makes glucose control more difficult.
   b. The combination of the work of labour together with hyperventilation due to pain rapidly leads to dehydration and ketosis. This is overcome by accurate fluid balance and adequate fluid replacement but ketosis is less likely to occur with effective epidural analgesia.
   c. Operative delivery is more likely and can usually be performed under the cover of epidural analgesia so avoiding the added hazards of general anaesthesia.

9. *Monitoring.* Electronic monitoring is mandatory. External monitoring should be commenced as soon as the patient arrives on the labour ward. The membranes should be ruptured as soon as the fetal head is engaged and the cervix is at least 4 cm dilated so that direct internal monitoring can be carried out. Interpretation of the fetal heart rate trace is as for labour in non-diabetic patients (see Section 15.4.1) and should be backed up with fetal blood sampling (Section 15.5).

10. *Augmentation.* Augmentation of contractions by means of a syntocinon infusion is indicated according to standard criteria (see Section 8.2). The solution containing the syntocinon should not contain dextrose.

11. *Second stage.* There is no contraindication to allowing time for the fetal head to descend and rotate in the second stage of labour (see Section 1.8) as long as the fetus is not asphyxiated and the mother has an effective epidural. The duration of pushing, however, should probably not exceed 30 min.

12. *Delivery.* The potential problems that surround delivery of a diabetic infant should be anticipated as follows:
   a. Ensure adequate analgesia in order that maternal co-operation is not lost.
   b. Summon the obstetric registrar early in the second stage. He/she should be present to interpret the fetal heart rate trace in the second stage and to act accordingly should there be fetal distress (see Section 15.4.1), shoulder dystocia (see Chapter 24) or other difficulty with delivery.

    c.   Summon the paediatrician in advance of the delivery.

    d.   Call the anaesthetist, who may remain outside the delivery room if there is an effective epidural.

    e.   Operative delivery is performed for standard indications only (see Chapter 26).

27.2.2 Elective deliveries

Diabetic patients should be admitted the night before planned delivery. They should receive their usual dose of insulin on the evening before induction together with an evening meal and a late snack if appropriate.

They should undergo the standard admission procedure (see Section 7.2) but, in addition, they should have a 30 min CTG which should be seen and signed by the duty registrar. Venous blood should be taken for:

1. Haemoglobin estimation.
2. Group and save serum (or cross-match two units if delivery is to be by elective Caesarean section).
3. Urea and electrolytes.

On the day of delivery the patient should omit breakfast and her morning dose of insulin and an infusion made up of 1 ℓ of 10 per cent dextrose with 30 units of soluble insulin and 2g KCl should be started at 0600 hours.

27.2.2.1 INDUCTION

Induction of labour should be by standard means (see Section 7.3) and should be started before 0700 hours. The patient should preferably be delivered in the same day. She should receive prophylaxis against Mendelson's syndrome as detailed in Section 3.8. If the patient has agreed to epidural analgesia it is unnecessary to wait until the patient is in labour before it is inserted. It will facilitate artificial rupture of the membranes, and if induction fails this will always result in Caesarean section in a diabetic patient and the epidural may be used to provide anaesthesia for the operation.

27.2.2.2 ELECTIVE CAESAREAN SECTION

This should be arranged with the duty anaesthetist the day before operation. The patient should be the first surgical case of the day. She should receive prophylaxis against Mendelson's syndrome as detailed in Section 3.8.

27.2.3 Management after delivery

1. The patient should remain on the labour ward until the next day.
2. The infusion of 10 per cent dextrose, insulin and KCl should be continued until the next day.
3. Capillary blood estimations should be made every 2 h if they are within the range of 5–10 mmol ℓ^{-1}. If not they should be made hourly and the infusion altered according to Table 27.1.

4. The next morning, if the patient has bowel sounds she should be started on a normal diet and given the same dose of insulin that she required before she became pregnant. If no bowel sounds are present she should continue on the above infusion until they return.

27.3 GESTATIONAL DIABETES

Gestational diabetes is strictly defined as abnormal or impaired glucose tolerance in pregnancy that returns to normal after delivery. As the patient's glucose tolerance following delivery is not yet known the following management applies to all patients who were not known to be diabetic before pregnancy.

27.3.1 Patients requiring insulin in pregnancy

These patients should be managed along the lines of insulin-dependent diabetics (see above). After delivery, however, their insulin requirements fall to zero and so they do not need to remain on insulin infusions. The infusion can be discontinued and the capillary blood testing should be stopped. A repeat glucose tolerance test should be arranged for six weeks after delivery to confirm the diagnosis of gestational diabetes.

27.3.2 Patients controlled on diet alone

These patients do not usually require insulin to cover labour and should be managed as follows:

1. Start an intravenous infusion of normal saline. Send venous blood for haemoglobin estimation and ask for serum to be saved.
2. Capillary blood glucose should be estimated by means of BM sticks or Dextrostix every 2 h. If the level exceeds 10 mmol ℓ^{-1} start an insulin infusion as detailed in Section 27.2 and manage the patient as though she was an insulin-dependent diabetic.
3. Take the same precautions for delivery as are detailed in Section 27.2.
4. If the patient has required insulin it may be stopped as soon as the delivery is over. Further capillary blood glucose estimations are also unnecessary.

27.4 NEONATAL CARE

Infants born to all mothers who have diabetes (insulin-dependent or gestational) are at risk from the complications detailed in Section 27.1. The infants should therefore *routinely* be sent to the neonatal, special (or intensive care) unit. Management is as follows:

1. As soon as the infant has been resuscitated (if necessary) it should be dried and placed under a radiant heater.
2. Perform a capillary blood glucose estimation by means of BM sticks or Dextrostix.

3. Give the baby a bottle of glucose and water or milk formula.
4. Repeat the capillary blood glucose estimations as follows:
    a. Hourly for 4 h.
    b. Every 2 h for the next 4 h.
    c. Every 4 h until it is 24 h old.
        More frequent testing will be required if the blood glucose is low or if the baby is jittery or has a convulsion.
5. Give i.v. dextrose (1 ml kg^{-1} of 50 per cent dextrose diluted 50:50 with water for injection) if the capillary sugar is less than 1 mol ℓ^{-1}. If this occurs a venous blood sugar should be sent to the laboratory as the Dextrostix are inaccurate at low values. However, do not wait for the result before giving the i.v. dextrose because if convulsions occur there is an increased risk of long term cerebral damage. Infants with capillary glucose levels of less than 2 mol ℓ^{-1} should be given a further feed.
6. If a vein cannot be located, give glucagon 0.03 mg kg^{-1} i.m.
7. The infant can usually be returned to its mother if it has not become hypoglycaemic by 12 h of age but glucose testing should continue for 24 h as detailed above.
8. Check the infant's calcium level in the second day of life.
9. Check the infant's bilirubin level on the third day of life.

27.5   CONTRACEPTION

The combined oral contraceptive pill decreases glucose tolerance in patients who have had abnormal glucose tolerance in pregnancy but its effect on insulin-dependent diabetics is less predictable. There is also theoretical risk of an increase in vascular disease in insulin-dependent diabetics taking the combined oral contraceptive pill. However, these risks have to be considered in the light of an unplanned pregnancy so the following guidelines are suggested:

1. Patients with insulin-dependent diabetes who have not completed their family should be put on the combined oral contraceptive pill (providing there are no other contraindications) until their family is complete. Sterilization should then be offered.
2. Patients who have abnormal glucose tolerance in pregnancy which returns to normal after delivery may be put on the combined oral contraceptive if there are no contraindications.
3. Patients who continue to have impaired glucose tolerance after delivery or who are unable to take the combined oral contraceptive should be offered the progesterone-only pill or an intra-uterine contraceptive device. The failure rate of the progesterone-only pill is higher than the combined oral contraceptive pill (six versus one per 100 woman years) and up to 50 per cent of women will have menstrual irregularities. If the intra-uterine contraceptive device is chosen it should be a plastic device (a Lippes' loop) as the copper devices rapidly become encrusted with sulphur and chloride in diabetics.
4. Patients who are prepared to use barrier methods should also be encouraged to use a spermicidal cream, to increase the contraceptive efficacy.

Chapter 28

Cardiac Disease

28.1   INTRODUCTION

The incidence of cardiac disease in women of child-bearing age is falling and now stands at about 1 per cent. The proportion of affected women with congenital heart disease is rising and it is now becoming increasingly common to see pregnant women with surgically corrected congenital cardiac lesions.

Pregnancy, and in particular, labour, imposes enormous demands upon the cardio-vascular system. The time of greatest risk for the woman with cardiac disease is labour and the immediate puerperium.

Women with severe cardiac disease tend to tolerate anaesthesia and surgery poorly. Vaginal delivery is usually preferable, with Caesarean section being performed mostly for obstetric reasons. However, if there is a significant risk that pulmonary oedema may develop during labour, elective Caesarean section under general anaesthesia may provide a safer alternative.

Women with cardiac disease will have been carefully monitored throughout their pregnancy, with care taken to prevent cardiac failure, infection and anaemia.

28.2 MANAGEMENT OF LABOUR

28.2.1 General aspects

The patient should be nursed in a sitting position since the increased cardiac output, consequent upon increased venous return in the supine position, may lead to respiratory and cardiac embarrassment.

1. Observations:
    a. General condition of patient.
    b. Pulse rate and rhythm.
    c. Blood pressure.
    d. Respiratory rate.
2. Frequency:
    a. At least every 15 min.

28.2.2 Pulmonary oedema

28.2.2.1 SIGNS AND SYMPTOMS

Acute left ventricular failure causes breathlessness and the patient will appear extremely distressed. There may also be wheezing due to bronchial oedema and a cough productive of pink frothy sputum.

The patient will appear pale, with cold, sweaty extremities due to vasoconstriction. This can cause an initial rise in blood pressure. The patient usually sits upright holding on to a firm structure and uses her accessory muscles of respiration.

On examination of the chest, widespread crackles will be heard over the lung fields on auscultation which persist after several deep breaths. A third heart sound (associated with rapid left ventricular filling) will be heard at the apex or with the patient in the left lateral position. When associated with a tachycardia this is termed a gallop rhythm.

28.2.2.2 INVESTIGATIONS

1. Chest X-ray (see Figure 11.3).
2. Electrocardiograph (ECG). An ECG does not show pathognomonic signs of heart failure but may demonstrate a dysrhythmia which may have precipitated failure.
3. Blood cultures. These should be undertaken in all patients with known valvular disease associated with fever, to exclude endocarditis.
4. Full blood count. A relatively mild anaemia may precipitate failure in patients with cardiac disease.
5. Electrolytes and serum proteins. The severe hypoalbuminaemia often seen in the pre-eclamptic patient may cause pulmonary oedema, if the patient has coexistent heart disease (see Section 11.11).

28.2.2.3 TREATMENT

1. The patient should be propped sitting up, if possible with the legs dependent. Oxygen should be administered via face mask at 4 ℓ min^{-1}.

2. Drugs
   a. Frusemide 40 mg intravenously. This drug alone may relieve the pulmonary oedema, within half an hour.
   b. Diamorphine 10 mg im or 2.5 mg iv.
   c. Intravenous aminophylline (to relieve wheezing) should not be given as it may induce dysrhythmias and aggravate the pulmonary oedema resulting in death.
   d. Digoxin is *never* indicated for acute pulmonary oedema and is probably only ever indicated to control dysrhythmias.
3. Enlist the help of a cardiologist.
4. Other measures (if the above measures fail to cause improvement).
   a. Alternate cuffing of the thighs with a sphygmomanometer cuff inflated to just above venous pressure, will effectively reduce venous return and reduce pulmonary venous congestion.
   b. Venesection, removing up to 500 ml blood, should be attempted if the above measures fail.
   c. In extreme situations, the patient may require intubation and positive pressure ventilation. This works by reducing the venous return (because of the positive pressure) and by aiding evaporation of lung fluid.

28.2.3   Dysrhythmias

Any suspected abnormality of pulse rate or rhythm should be investigated by means of a standard 12 lead ECG with a II lead rhythm strip, and management should always be with the help of a cardiologist. The following guidelines are provided for urgent situations and to allow obstetricians to explain the likely course of action to their patients.

28.2.3.1   NORMAL

The pulse rate is increased by an average of 10 beats min^{-1} in pregnancy to a mean of about 80 beats min^{-1}. Premature atrial beats and ventricular ectopic beats are common in normal pregnancy and are suspected by an occasional dropped beat at the radial pulse.

The following abnormalities may occur: (see also Table 28.1).

Paroxysmal supraventricular tachycardia (SVT)

Pregnancy increases the number of attacks of SVT and some patients only have SVTs when they are pregnant.

In the absence of organic heart disease SVTs are usually readily controlled and rarely cause heart failure. Most patients with a long history of SVTs are able to stop them by means of the Valsalva manoeuvre or carotid sinus pressure and rarely attend hospital.

Patients with organic heart disease may go into heart failure within a few hours of SVT. The Valsalva manoeuvre may be tried but if carotid sinus massage is attempted it should be under ECG monitoring as ventricular extrasystoles or even ventricular fibrillation may occur.

If the above measures fail give 5 mg practolol slowly iv and repeat 30 min later if no effect is obtained. The fetal heart rate should be monitored in pregnancy of more

Table 28.1   Treatment of dysrhythmias presenting in patients in labour

Dysrhythmia	Therapy	Comment
1. Paroxysmal supraventricular tachycardia	Carotid sinus massage	With ECG monitoring
	No further therapy in absence of organic heart disease and/or symptoms	
	5 mg practalol iv × 2 doses	Monitor fetus
	50 mg phenytoin iv	
	DC shock	Care needed if patient is digitalized
2. Atrial fibrillation	0.25 mg digoxin every 8 h	To control ventricular rate
	Anticoagulate	
3. Atrial flutter	DC shock	
4. Ventricular tachycardia	100 mg lignocaine iv followed by 1 mg min^{-1}	
	DC shock and lignocaine (as above)	Following a myocardial infarction
5. Ventricular fibrillation	DC shock	
6. Complete heart block	None	If asymptomatic
	Pacing	If symptomatic

than 26 weeks gestation as practolol occasionally causes bradycardia.

If practolol fails (rarely) 50 mg phenytoin should be given iv. The alternative is direct current shock (200 joules) and this has been used in pregnancy without reported complications.

Atrial fibrillation (AF)

This is usually only seen in pregnancy with advanced mitral valve disease of rheumatic origin. It usually occurs in the second half of pregnancy and may occur for the first time in labour.

This requires *urgent* treatment because of the risks of heart failure and of arterial embolization. Start oral digoxin 0.25 mg every 8 h for 24–48 h (until the ventricular rate is controlled) and then give an appropriate maintenance dose. In view of the risks of arterial emboli the patient should be anticoagulated with 40 000 u heparin per day given by continuous intravenous infusion.

Patients with long standing AF who have a stable cardiac state and a controlled ventricular rate rarely develop problems in labour and no attempt should be made to restore sinus rhythm, as this may precipitate arterial embolisation.

Atrial flutter

This is rare in pregnancy and rarely occurs for the first time in labour. Its complications are as for atrial fibrillation but the treatment of choice is DC shock.

Ventricular tachycardia (VT)

This is a very rare complication of labour but requires prompt treatment.

Unless the patient has clear evidence of a myocardial infarction give 100 mg lignocaine as an iv bolus followed by 1 mg min^{-1} as a continuous infusion. Long term management will probably be with the newer anti-arrhythmic drugs such as amiodarone.

If the patient has had a myocardial infarction and is in heart failure because of the VT, DC shock followed by i.v. lignocaine is the treatment of choice.

Ventricular fibrillation (VF)

This will respond only to DC shock and the energy level should start at 400 joules.

Complete heart block

This may occur for the first time in labour in women with viral carditis or chronic rheumatic disease. Most patients are asymptomatic and require no treatment. If the patient has Stokes–Adams attacks or develops heart failure she will need a permanent pacemaker. Pregnancy outcome does not appear to be affected by pacing.

28.2.4   Analgesia

It is important to provide adequate analgesia during labour for these patients, to allay maternal anxiety and its associated tachycardia.

Epidural analgesia is the most efficient form of pain relief, and as it reduces venous return by sympathetic blockade and peripheral vasodilation it will reduce cardiac output. Epidural analgesia is *positively contraindicated* in conditions which rely on venous return for an adequate cardiac output:

1.   Hypertrophic obstructive cardiomyopathy.
2.   Aortic stenosis.
3.   Eisenmenger's syndrome.

28.2.5   Prevention of infective endocarditis

Prophylactic antibiotic therapy is advised to cover labour in patients with rheumatic valvular disease, (particularly aortic incompetence and mitral incompetence), artificial valve prostheses or congenital heart disease. Infection is particularly likely if instrumental or surgical delivery is necessary.

The following three antibiotics are given commencing at the time of spontaneous or artificial rupture of the membranes and are continued until one dose after delivery.

Drug and dose:

1. Ampicillin 500 mg iv every 6 h.
2. Gentamicin 80 mg iv every 8 h.
3. Metronidazole 500 mg iv every 8 h.

or

4. Vancomycin 500 mg iv as a single dose (in place of ampicillin if the patient is penicillin-sensitive).

If the patient is to be delivered by elective Caesarean section the above drugs need to be given 1 h before surgery only.

28.2.6   Anticoagulation

Full anticoagulation with warfarin therapy during pregnancy is essential in patients with severe mitral valve disease, pulmonary valve disease, artificial valve replacements, atrial fibrillation or Eisenmenger's syndrome.

At about 37 weeks' gestation, the patient should be admitted to hospital, and commenced on full dose intravenous heparin, 40 000 i.u. per day should be administered by means of an infusion pump. If possible the heparin level should be assayed by means of protamine sulphate neutralization which should be maintained at 0.4–0.6 units per ml.

This regimen is continued until seven days postpartum, after which the risk of bleeding from the genital tract is reduced, when warfarin can be recommenced. If labour begins before 37 weeks whilst the patient is taking warfarin, vitamin K (Phytomenadione) is administered to the patient, the warfarin is discontinued and intravenous heparin commenced as above. A slow intravenous injection of 2.5 mg phytomenadione is given and the prothrombin time measured 3 h later. If the response is inadequate, the dose may be repeated. Phytomenadione will take up to 12 h to act and will prevent oral anticoagulants from acting for several days or even weeks.

28.2.7   Preterm labour

The use of β-sympathomimetic drugs, such as ritodrine, either alone or, in particular, in conjunction with corticosteroids, is to be avoided in the cardiac patient. This is because of both the direct chronotropic effect (β-1 agonist) and the reflex tachycardia as a result of vasodilation (β-2 agonist). Corticosteroids enhance this effect by their mineralocorticoid action leading to an increased circulatory volume, and hypokalaemia, leading to further myocardial impairment and the possibility of toxicity if digoxin is being used.

28.3   SECOND AND THIRD STAGES OF LABOUR

28.3.1   Patients with mild cardiac disease

These patients should be allowed to attempt a normal delivery if they have no basal crepitations at the onset of the second stage; i.m. syntometrine may be given as usual.

Table 28.2   Drug therapy and breast feeding

Drug	Excreted in breast milk	Effect on infant
Coumarin anticoagulants e.g. warfarin	Yes (small amounts)	Monitor infant by prothrombin time
Digoxin	Yes	Unlikely to affect in therapeutic doses
Frusemide	Not detected	—
Heparin	Not detected	Destroyed by alimentary system
Inanedione anticoagulants e.g. phenindione	Yes	Contraindicated
Phytomenadione (Vit K_1)	Small amounts	Unlikely to affect infant in therapeutic doses

28.3.2   Patients with latent/frank pulmonary oedema

Patients with crepitations should not be allowed to push and should undergo elective instrumental delivery. However, this should be an outlet forceps (or Ventouse delivery). There is no contraindication to allowing the head to descend in the second stage as long as the patient has adequate analgesia, which effectively means epidural analgesia.

Ergometrine (and syntometrine) should be avoided and ten units of syntocinon i.v. should be given with the delivery of the anterior shoulder.

28.4   BREAST FEEDING

If the patient wishes to breast feed she should be encouraged to do so unless she is on a drug which precludes it (see Table 28.2).

Chapter 29

Sickle Cell Disease and the Haemoglobinopathies

29.1   INTRODUCTION

Women with homozygous sickle cell disease (SS) and other compound heterozygotes for haemoglobin variants, e.g. SC disease and SThal, suffer increased maternal and fetal risk during pregnancy.

Sickle cell haemoglobin is the commonest structural variant of the globin chain and results in distortion of the red cell when the haemoglobin is in its reduced form. Sickled red cells are relatively rigid, and block small blood vessels. Sickle cells also have a shortened survival. A haemoglobin concentration of at least 7 g dl^{-1} is maintained by increased erythropoiesis. This leads to increased folate requirements, therefore supplements should be routine antenatally.

Homozygous sickle cell anaemia (SS disease) is characterized by periods of relative well-being interrupted by episodes of acute sickling of red cells known as crises. Sickling crises results in progressive organ damage, as a result of tissue infarction due to vascular occlusion. Vascular occlusion itself tends to encourage further sickling.

Women with HbSS and HbSThal have similar clinical features, and although HbSC disease is a milder variant, serious sickling crises are particularly common in pregnancy and the puerperium.

29.2 PREGNANCY IN SICKLE CELL DISEASE

The woman with sickle cell disease may embark on pregnancy with evidence of previous organ damage due to the disease. This may include:

1. Pelvic arthropathy with avascular necrosis of the femoral head.
2. Chronic renal failure.

There is an over-all fetal loss of about 45 per cent due to:

1. Spontaneous abortion.
2. Intra-uterine growth retardation.
3. Preterm delivery.

The maternal mortality is about 6 per cent, and mainly secondary to cardiac failure from severe anaemia and thromboembolic complications. Maternal complications associated with pregnancy include:

1. Upper urinary tract infections.
2. Pulmonary infections, particularly pneumococcal pneumonia.
3. Salmonella.
4. Puerperal endometritis.
5. An increased risk of pre-eclampsia.

29.3 SICKLE CELL CRISIS

This is characterized by severe abdominal and/or bone pain and is accompanied by fever and a leucocytosis, with hepatosplenomegaly.
Precipitating factors include:

1. Hypoxia.
2. Metabolic acidosis.
3. Dehydration.
4. Extremes of temperature.
5. Infection.

29.3.1 Management of a sickle cell crisis

Avoidance of known precipitating factors (see above) will reduce the likelihood of a crisis. The aims of treatment of a sickle crisis are to reverse the causal factors.

29.3.2 Investigations

1. Hb, differential white cell count, haematocrit.
2. Blood group and save serum.
3. Liver function tests.
4. Urea and electrolytes.
5. Arterial blood gases.
6. Infection screen.
    a. Mid-stream specimen of urine.
    b. Blood culture.
    c. Sputum for culture and detection of fat cells (to detect bone marrow embolism).
7. Chest X-ray (if applicable).
8. Strict fluid balance recordings should take place.

29.3.3 Treatment

1. Rest.
2. Warmth: the patient should be kept comfortably warm but not overheated.
3. Analgesia.
4. Rehydration: $3 \ \ell$ fluid m^{-2} of body area (about $4 \ \ell$ day^{-1} should be given every 24 h). Crystalloid solutions or fresh frozen plasma can be used, and oral fluid intake is encouraged to maintain hydration as above.
5. Oxygen by face mask.
6. Appropriate treatment of infection, having identified the site, causal organisms and antibiotic sensitivity.
7. Transfusion. This can be in the form of:
    a. Partial exchange.
    b. Exchange.

    Some authors advocate repeated transfusions of three to four units of blood in the pregnant woman with sickle cell disease, commencing at booking, and repeated every six weeks in order to maintain a level of HbS of less than 10 per cent, and a haemoglobin concentration of 10.5–12.5 g dl^{-1}. This is thought to reduce the erythropoietic stimulus to the bone marrow, reduce the chances of sickle crises, and improve fetal outlook.

    However, repeated transfusions carry significant risks to the individual of:
    a. Immunological reactions.
    b. Potassium and calcium disturbances.
    c. Transmission of viruses such as hepatitis B and HIV.
    d. Red cell antigen immunization which may lead to difficulty in subsequent cross-matching.
    e. The development of anti-Duffy, anti-Lewis and antibodies to the MNS system which may cross the placenta and result in isoimmunization and haemolytic disease of the new born.

    A prophylactic repeated transfusion regime has yet to be fully evaluated as the correct routine for management of these patients in pregnancy.

29.3.4   Exchange transfusion

Exchange transfusion is recommended in the sickle cell crisis when the haemoglobin concentration falls to less than 6 g dl⁻¹ or at a rate of 2 g or more per 24 h.

1. Give 1 ℓ of normal saline via a 16 gauge cannula. Set up a further litre of saline in order to keep the vein open.
2. Have the cross-matched, whole blood ready.
3. Using 50 ml (or 100 ml) syringes remove 500 ml from the other arm via an in-dwelling 16 gauge cannula, kept patent with heparin (10 u ml⁻¹).
4. Give one unit of blood via the cannula receiving saline.
5. Remove and exchange one blood volume. If the haemoglobin is less than 8 g dl⁻¹ (with more than 40 per cent HbS) give five additional units, aiming for a final haemoglobin of about 12 g dl⁻¹.
6. Venesection usually becomes easier after two to three units but exchange may take two days.
7. Keep accurate fluid balance records. Observe pulse and BP hourly together with conscious state. A deterioration may suggest CNS sludging and fluid intake should be increased.
8. Do not give diuretics.
9. Give 4 ℓ normal saline a day during the exchange.
10. Give 600 mg benzylpenicillin i.m. every 6 h to reduce the likelihood of overwhelming pneumococcus infection. Treat other infections as appropriate.

29.4   MANAGEMENT OF LABOUR

The following are suggested guidelines.

29.4.1   Investigations

1. Hb, haematocrit.
2. Grouping and cross-matching of two units of blood.

   Both these investigations should be performed when the patient first enters the labour ward, since there may be delay in cross-matching due to irregular antibodies induced by repeated transfusions.

29.4.2   Analgesia

Ensure adequate analgesia with following precautions:

1. Epidural. Epidural block is not favoured, because of the vascular stasis induced by venous pooling as a result of sympathetic blockade, which may encourage sickling.

2. Entonox. Entonox may be beneficial and has the added advantage of simultaneously providing 50 per cent oxygen.
3. Narcotic analgesics. Pethidine may be used; there are no particular contraindications.

29.4.3   Other measures

1. No tourniquets should be used during venepuncture or exchange transfusions.
2. Fluids. Input and output should be accurately recorded. Intravenous Hartmann's solution during labour should be administered at a minimum rate of 1 ℓ every 3 h.
3. Humidified facial oxygen should be administered from the time analgesia is given.
4. Warmth should be ensured by keeping the room temperature at about 20 °C.
5. Inform anaesthetic and paediatric staff when labour has been diagnosed. The anaesthetist will then be able to see the patient and her notes in case she requires his/her services later. The paediatrician may wish to sample the cord blood in order to determine whether the fetus is going to suffer from sickle cell disease or trait. Babies with sickle cell disease do not have complications in the first three months of life as haemoglobin F still predominates.
6. If general anaesthesia is necessary, antibiotic prophylaxis (600 mg benzylpenicillin i.m. 6 hourly) should be given.
7. Humidified facial oxygen should be continued for the first 12 hours after delivery.

29.5   THE PUERPERIUM

The patient should be kept warm and well hydrated. Folic acid supplements should continue for 6 weeks.

The combined oral contraceptive is best avoided. Depot-progestogens are the commonly advised form of contraception as there is some evidence that it reduces the number of crises.

29.6   SICKLE CELL TRAIT

These patients do not suffer from any particular complications in pregnancy, but hypoxia and dehydration should be avoided during anaesthesia and labour, and in the immediate puerperium. Epidural analgesia carries no additional risks.

Chapter 30

Australia Antigen Positive Patients

30.1 INTRODUCTION

Many antenatal patients are being routinely tested at booking for the presence of hepatitis antigens. The screening test will identify those women who are surface antigen (Australia antigen) positive (HB_sAg positive). In these women, the sample is further tested to determine whether they are carriers of the e antigen and the anti-e antibody.

For the purposes of the risk of infectivity to attending staff, however, all surface antigen positive women should be treated alike, regardless of the e antigen/antibody results, although it is recognized that the risks of infection are different. There are also differing consequences for the fetus, as the vertical transmission risk varies according to the e antigen status.

Most infective: HB$_e$Ag positive ± anti-HB$_e$ negative
Least infective: HB$_s$Ag negative and anti-HB$_e$ positive

All women who are HB$_s$Ag positive carry a risk of transmission of the virus, which is secreted in all body fluids. Extreme care must therefore be taken when managing these women in labour, for the protection of the staff and other patients.

Warning labels marked 'Australia antigen' in the form of yellow stickers should be used liberally in suspected or proven cases.

30.2   HIGH RISK CATEGORIES

The following patients are at a high risk of being Australia antigen positive and all samples sent to the laboratory should be marked with a yellow sticker until their Australia antigen status is known. If negative the stickers should be removed from the notes.

1. Patients with acute or chronic liver disease.
2. Patients who have been treated at any time in a renal dialysis unit.
3. Patients who have received five or more units of blood in the past.
4. All patients that have had any blood transfusions in the tropics or sub-tropics.
5. All patients who have lived in areas outside North West Europe, North America, Australia or New Zealand.
6. Drug addicts.
7. Homosexuals.
8. Prostitutes.
9. Patients with extensive tattooing.
10. Patients with Down's syndrome.
11. Patients with polyarteritis nodosa.

30.3   MANAGEMENT IN LABOUR

30.3.1   Equipment

Where possible all equipment used to deal with Australia antigen positive patients should be disposable. The woman should be nursed in isolation during labour and the usual rules for isolation should be followed.

30.3.2   General guidelines

1. All specimens should be placed in a sealed container which should then be placed in a self-seal plastic bag which must have a yellow label on the outside.
2. The request form (which must also have a yellow label) *must not* be enclosed with the specimen but should be in the outside pocket of a self-seal plastic bag.
3. Staff with cuts or abrasions should not attend Australia antigen positive patients.

30.3.3   Suspected cases

1. A yellow label should be attached to the case notes and to the bed notes.
2. Blood specimens should be tested immediately.
3. The yellow labels should be removed later if the test is negative.

30.3.4   Positive cases

1. Australia antigen positive women must be nursed in a side room whenever possible.
2. Procedures involving puncture of the woman's skin should be kept to a minimum. Members of staff giving injections or taking bloods should wear two pairs of disposable gloves as well as mask and gown.
3. Members of staff who are splashed by any exudate from the patient should wash the area immediately and the procedure for accidental contamination (see Section 30.4) should be followed.
4. Linen. Disposable items should be used where possible and placed in the appropriate bag for burning. Contaminated non-disposable items should be placed in appropriately colour-coded bags. Where there is excessive blood loss disposable linen must be used.
5. Equipment. Non-metallic and non-disposable items should be immersed in 1 per cent sodium hypochlorite solution for 30 min (that is 10 000 parts per million of available chlorine). Metallic objects should be immersed in 2 per cent glutaraldehyde for 30 min or autoclaved if possible.
6. Sharps. All syringes, needles and sharps including glass ampoules, scalpel blades, razor blades, suture cutters and needles should be placed in the appropriate container immediately after use.
7. Urine and faeces should be covered with 1 per cent sodium hypochlorite solution and disposed of at once. Care should be taken to avoid splashing.
8. Splashes. If blood, faeces or any exudate is spilt on any surface it should be carefully wiped away and the surface washed with 1 per cent sodium hypochlorite solution.
9. Placentae. These should be double-wrapped in plastic bags and incinerated.

30.4   ACCIDENTAL CONTAMINATION

Hepatitis B virus is present in all body fluids of infected patients and may be transmitted when such body fluid comes into contact with fresh cuts or abrasions in the skin or mucus membrane or when the virus is accidentally inoculated by means of a sharp instrument.

Any person who undergoes accidental exposure should carry out the following procedure:

1. Wash the area well and treat any cuts or needle stabs with alcohol.
2. Report the accident to your superior who should then send you to the occupational health department or to casualty.

3. Blood samples from the patient and from yourself should be sent to the virology department.
4. The public health (or virology) laboratory will decide whether you should receive immunoglobulin. Where possible this should be given within 48 h but certainly should be given no later than ten days. A second dose is usually given at one month.

30.5 PATIENTS FOR THEATRE

In some hospitals a specific operating theatre is set aside for use for Australia antigen positive patients. If not try to use a theatre that does not need to be used again immediately.

30.5.1 Collection of patient for theatre

The linen on the trolley should be disposable. If the patient is bleeding or if there is other exudate present then gowns and disposable gloves should be worn to move the patient to theatre.

30.5.2 The anaesthetic room

1. The anaesthetist and nurse should wear disposable masks, gowns, gloves and over-shoes.
2. All staff should wear disposable theatre wear including gowns and overshoes over theatre boots.
3. Unscrubbed staff should wear disposable gowns, gloves and plastic aprons. Scrubbed staff should wear disposable gowns, caps, masks and plastic aprons. Disposable drapes should be used wherever possible.
4. Swabs should be counted onto a plastic sheet on the floor and not onto the swab rack.
5. Use disposable scalpels where possible. If disposable scalpels are not available the scalpel should be decontaminated by 2 per cent glutaraldehyde for at least 30 min before blades are removed. As an alternative the scalpels may be autoclaved.
6. The sucker bottles should be filled half full with 1 per cent sodium hypochlorite solution.
7. Decontamination
   a. 1 per cent sodium hypochlorite should be used for non-metallic items.
   b. 2 per cent glutaraldehyde should be used for metallic instruments, trolleys, operating tables and theatre in general.
   c. All instruments should be heat-sterilized whenever possible.

30.5.3 Recovery

The patient should be recovered in theatre if possible.

30.5.4 Return to the ward

The theatre nurse must ensure that the patient's skin is completely clean from blood and other exudate. The patient should wear a clean disposable operating gown.

30.5.5 Operation procedure

The names of all staff present should be recorded. Details of any injury or splash should also be recorded.

30.6 THE BABY

The mothers who are at most risk of infecting their babies are those who are HB_cAg positive. After delivery the baby should be given an injection of hepatitis B immunoglobulin and vaccinated against hepatitis. 0.5 ml vaccine should be given immediately, at six weeks and at three months. This will protect most infants but a few may still develop hepatitis B, as transplacental infection has been described. Those infants that are affected are at long term risk of chronic active hepatitis and hepatocellular carcinoma.

Mothers who are surface antigen positive may be allowed to breast feed. Even though the virus is excreted in the breast milk, prohibiting breast feeding does not stop transmission as it occurs via saliva during kissing.

Chapter 31

The Acquired Immunodeficiency Syndrome (AIDS)

31.1   INTRODUCTION

In 1983 a new virus was discovered which was identified as the vector of the acquired immunodeficiency syndrome (AIDS). Formerly named human T-lymphotropic virus 3 (HTLV3) it is now known as human immunodeficiency virus or HIV. The prevalence of AIDS in the UK is four per million (at the time of writing) being far more common in men than women.

HIV infection can be acquired by normal vaginal intercourse, anal intercourse, parenteral drug abuse when needles are shared, Factor VIII concentrates which have not been heat-treated, infected blood transfusions, donor organ transplantation, and by vertical transmission from mother to fetus.

The mortality is 80 per cent at two years.

The significance of HIV infection in obstetrics is that:

1. At-risk groups of women (see Table 31.1) should be identified and screened for antibody status.
2. Vertical transmission to the fetus does occur.
3. Special precautions should be taken on the labour ward to protect staff and other patients.

31.2   SCREENING

Tests for HIV antibodies are available and have a very low false positive rate. Seroconverison, however, may take 1–8 weeks. Positive tests should be repeated for

Table 31.1   Groups in the Western World at potential risk of HIV infection

1. Parenteral drug abusers (these comprise >40 per cent women known to be HIV positive).
2. Sexual partners of parenteral drug abusers.
3. Haemophiliacs
4. Sexual partners of haemophiliacs
5. Persons of Central African origin, (Burundi, Congo, Kenya, Rwanda, Tanzania, Uganda, Zaire, Zambia) or who have been resident, or whose sexual partners have been resident in Central African countries for more than six months in the last six years.
6. Renal transplant recipients (before 1985).
7. Prostitutes.
8. Breast-fed infants of infected mothers.
9. Sexual partners of homosexual and bisexual men.

Table 31.2   Features of acute HIV infection

Glandular-fever-like illness
Fevers
Sweats
Malaise
Anorexia
Generalized aches and pains
Diarrhoea
Macular rash
Lymphadenopathy
Acute encephalopathy
Acute neuropathy
Mood and personality changes
Epileptic fits
Coma

confirmation. Screening is justified in the at-risk groups listed in Table 31.1, and in women with suspected acute HIV infection (see Table 31.2). Routine screening is controversial and is not practised at present.

31.3   VERTICAL TRANSMISSION

HIV is transmissible to the fetus *in utero*. The fetus has a two in three chance of infection if the mother is seropositive, and a 50 per cent risk of death if it is infected. The seropositive woman herself is at greater risk of developing clinical disease during pregnancy than when she is not pregnant, possibly due to depression of lymphocyte responsiveness.

Preterm delivery and IUGR commonly occur in seropositive women. There may be neonatal hepatosplenomegaly, and by the age of six months the infant exhibits:

1. Failure to thrive.
2. Recurrent fevers.

3. Respiratory disease.
4. Lymphadenopathy.

If a seropositive patient presents in early pregnancy termination may be justified.

31.4 SPECIAL PRECAUTIONS DURING LABOUR

The risk to hospital staff is very low, and less than the quoted one in four risk of acquiring hepatitis B following a needle injury. AIDS has not been described in any health care worker as a result of accidental exposure. The risk to other labouring women in the same unit is negligible. The concentration of HIV in body fluid is very low except in blood.

Table 31.3 illustrates the guidelines to follow in labour for seropositive women.

Table 31.3   Management of HIV-positive women in labour and after delivery

1. General precautions as for hepatitis-B-positive women (see Section 30.3).
2. Steroids are contraindicated.
3. Continuous external FHRM should be used.
4. FSE, FBS are contraindicated.
5. Operative delivery is indicated for the usual reasons (see Section 26.2), but avoid the Ventouse.
6. Episiotomy as required.
7. Placentae should be examined in the delivery room and then incinerated.
8. The paediatrician should be present at delivery (baby may have IUGR, be preterm and/or suffer narcotic withdrawal).
9. Wash and examine the baby in the delivery room.
10. Single postnatal room with en-suite bathroom and toilet.
11. Breast-feeding does carry a small risk to an uninfected infant, and therefore is contraindicated.
12. Avoid live vaccines in childhood.

31.5 LEGAL ASPECTS

The patient who refuses to be screened must have her wishes respected. Strict confidentiality should surround seropositive patients, because if their seropositivity is discovered this may have profound social consequences, and she may be unable to obtain insurance, a mortgage and even a job without illegally denying her seropositivity.

The patient in an at-risk group who refuses the screening test should be managed as though she was seropositive.

Doctors and midwives have no right to refuse to care for seropositive patients.

II

COMPLICATED LABOUR

C. Special Situations

Chapter 32

Trial of Labour

32.1 Introduction
32.2 Conducting a trial of labour
32.3 Subsequent pregnancies

32.1 INTRODUCTION

The term 'trial of labour' is usually reserved for patients in whom there is an antenatal suspicion that the mother may have a small pelvis for that particular baby. The following patients may have a small pelvis:

1. Women under 5 feet (152 cm) tall who have a shoe size of three or less. These women often have a small gynaecoid pelvis.
2. Patients with a high head at term, in whom there is no other obvious cause.

Unless there is a history of trauma to the pelvis, rickets or pelvic tuberculosis, performing erect lateral pelvimetry in late pregnancy or early labour is unhelpful in predicting whether vaginal delivery will be possible. Unless the pelvis is grossly distorted by the above conditions all patients should be allowed a trial of labour.

32.2 CONDUCTING A TRIAL OF LABOUR

1. It is preferable to await the spontaneous onset of labour as this gives the patient her best chance of a vaginal delivery. Induction of labour fails in at least 5 per cent of patients and the argument for induction at 38 weeks in order to prevent further head growth and hardening of the fetal skull is fallacious. Fetal head growth effectively stops after 37 weeks gestation and moulding occurs even in postmature infants.
2. If a patient is admitted in labour with a high head the following factors must be excluded before conducting a trial of labour:
    a. Placenta praevia.
    b. A fetal abnormality, e.g. hydrocephaly.
    c. A pelvic tumour.

    d. A malpresentation (see Chapter 20).

If these factors have not been excluded antenatally a real time scan may be performed on the labour ward.

3. Start an infusion of normal saline through a cannula of at least 16 gauge and send blood for:
   a. Haemoglobin estimation.
   b. Serum to be saved.
4. Start prophylaxis against Mendelson's syndrome as detailed in Section 3.8.
5. Perform an abdominal palpation on admission and then every hour so that the descent of the fetal head may be followed by means of the system of fifths palpable (see Section 1.4).
6. Provide adequate analgesia, a constant attendant and continuous electronic fetal monitoring.
7. Perform a vaginal examination on admission to confirm labour, to exclude a malpresentation (see Chapter 20) and to note the cervical dilatation. *Do not* rupture the membranes until the fetal head is at least fixed in the pelvic brim.
8. If the membranes rupture spontaneously and the fetal head is still high perform an immediate vaginal examination to exclude a cord prolapse.
9. Repeat the vaginal examination every 3 h and if the rate of cervical dilatation falls 2 h or more to the right of the line of expected progress (see Section 1.4) the following guidelines should be applied:
   a. If the fetal head is fixed in the pelvic brim (or engaged) perform an ARM. If necessary use an assistant to apply gentle pressure to the uterine fundus to prevent the fetal head being pushed up. After the amniotic fluid has escaped the head should settle into the pelvis. Apply a fetal scalp electrode if possible. Wait 2 h and if the contractions are not moderate to strong and occurring every 3 min or less start an infusion of syntocinon as detailed in Section 7.3.3. Lack of progress can be confirmed by performing a vaginal examination at this stage.
   b. If the membranes cannot be ruptured start the syntocinon infusion and re-examine the patient after 3 h on full dose syntocinon. If the membranes cannot be ruptured at this time perform a Caesarean section.
10. Manage dysfunctional labour as detailed in Section 8.2.
11. Caesarean section is indicated for the following reasons:
   a. Fetal distress. If the fetal head is still high and a serious abnormality (see Section 15.4) of the fetal heart rate trace occurs it is usually necessary to perform a Caesarean section because fetal blood sampling will not be possible.
   b. Cord prolapse.
   c. Failure to be able to rupture the membranes after 3 h on full dose (40 mu min^{-1}) syntocinon.
   d. Prolonged latent phase (PLP) unresponsive to syntocinon (see Section 8.2).
   e. Secondary arrest of cervical dilatation (SACD) that fails to respond to syntocinon (see Section 8.2).

It should be obvious from the above reasons for Caesarean section that all labours (especially in primigravidae) are best regarded as 'trials of labour'.

32.3   SUBSEQUENT PREGNANCIES

A patient who has undergone a Caesarean section for a failed trial of labour managed as detailed above should have an elective Caesarean section at 38 weeks in the next and all subsequent pregnancies.

Chapter 33
Trial of Scar

33.1 INTRODUCTION

A trial of scar is performed when the patient has a uterine scar as a result of previous surgery or following a Caesarean section for a non-recurring cause.

33.2 CONTRAINDICATIONS

1. Classical Caesarean section scar. If the patient has had a vertical uterine incision that extends to or over the uterine fundus she should be delivered by elective Caesarean section (lower segment) at 37–38 weeks gestation in all subsequent pregnancies. If the patient has had a lower vertical uterine incision (De Lee incision) a trial of scar in the next pregnancy is reasonable.
2. An extensive myomectomy, particularly if the uterine cavity has been opened. This is said to weaken the uterus.
3. A recurring cause for Caesarean section, for example cephalo-pelvic disproportion.
4. An obstetric reason for Caesarean section in this pregnancy, for example, placenta praevia.

33.3 CONDUCTING A TRIAL OF SCAR

1. It is preferable to await the onset of spontaneous labour if possible as this removes the added hazard of a failed induction. If induction of labour is necessary, repeated prostaglandin pessaries should be used with caution (see Section 23.3).
2. On admission review the history and ensure that the trial of scar is appropriate.
3. Start an infusion of normal saline through a cannula of at least 16 gauge. Send venous blood for haemoglobin and ask for the serum to be saved.

4. Perform a vaginal examination and rupture the membranes if the fetal head is engaged and the cervix is 4 cm or more dilated.

5. Provide a constant attendant and continuous electronic fetal heart rate monitoring.

6. Analgesia. Provide adequate analgesia. Epidural anaesthesia does not mask rupture of a uterine scar. An incomplete rupture is usually painless because the scar is composed of fibrous tissue which is not innervated. If, however, a woman with an effective epidural complains of pain she should be examined carefully to exclude a complete rupture of the uterus (see Section 23.4). In this situation the pain arises from generalized peritoneal irritation.

7. Augmentation. If cervical dilatation falls 2 h or more to the right of the line of expected progress (see Section 1.4) the patient should be examined to exclude a malpresentation (see Chapter 20) and then labour may be augmented by using a solution of 5 i.u. of syntocinon in 1 ℓ of normal saline (see Section 7.3.3). A repeat vaginal examination should be performed after 3 h of syntocinon at 80 drops min^{-1} (20 mu min^{-1}) and if there has been no further cervical dilatation a Caesarean section should be performed. In this situation intra-uterine pressure monitoring may be helpful (see Section 7.4).

8. Post delivery. Some obstetricians advocate feeling the uterine scar to determine if it is intact. This is not sound advice for the following reasons:

   a. An epidural or general anaesthetic is required to properly examine the scar.

   b. The examiner may convert an incomplete uterine rupture to a complete rupture (see Section 23.2).

   c. If the uterus is well contracted following delivery and there is no significant vaginal bleeding uterine rupture is very unlikely.

Chapter 34

The Obstetric Flying Squad

34.1   Introduction

34.2   Personnel

34.3   Procedure and equipment

34.1   INTRODUCTION

The obstetric flying squad exists to manage patients who are thought by their general practitioner, midwife, district nurse or the ambulance man to be more at risk by being transported to hospital than by awaiting the flying squad. Such circumstances are as follows:

1.   Retained placenta.
2.   Severe APH.
3.   Postabortal bleeding.
4.   Imminent delivery.

34.2   PERSONNEL

The team consists of the:

1.   Duty obstetric registrar.
2.   A senior midwife.

In addition it may be appropriate to take:

3.   A paediatrician.
4.   An anaesthetist.

34.3   PROCEDURE AND EQUIPMENT

On no account should a flying squad call ever be refused and there is rarely a case for attempting diagnosis and management at the end of a telephone.

1. Telephone calls requesting the obstetric flying squad are usually put through to the labour ward and should be dealt with by a senior midwife.
2. Record the following information:
    a. Name, address and telephone number (if appropriate) of the woman.
    b. Name and designation of the person requesting the flying squad.
    c. The reason for the request.
3. Procedures for arranging the flying squad ambulance vary locally and will either be:
    a. The labour ward has the telephone number of the local ambulance service and summons an ambulance.
    b. The person attending the patient summons an ambulance or directs the ambulance that is present to the hospital to pick up the flying squad.
4. Before leaving the hospital the duty registrar should inform his/her direct superior that he/she is going on a flying squad call and request him/her to come in to cover the labour ward. In some hospitals there is an arrangement whereby the senior goes on the flying squad call directly from home. *The labour ward must not be left uncovered.*
5. The members of the flying squad should collect the following equipment:
    a. Two units of O negative blood and an insulated box in which to transport them. This blood should be kept close to the labour ward and must be kept constantly up to date.
    b. A prepared box of emergency drugs (Table 34.1).
    c. A prepared delivery pack (Table 34.2).
    d. A prepared neonatal resuscitation pack (Table 34.3).
    e. A portable drip stand.
    f. A cylinder of Entonox.
7. On arrival at the patient's house the registrar should make a rapid assessment of the situation. It is often possible to perform initial resuscitative measures and then transport the patient back to hospital. This is not appropriate in the following circumstances:
    a. Retained placenta. After initial resuscitation it is safer to perform a manual removal in the woman's home as moving her will often start torrential bleeding.

Table 34.1 Drugs for use by the flying squad

Drug	Amount
Syntometrine	3 ampoules
Ergometrine	2×0.5 mg
Syntocinon	5×5 i.u.
Pethidine	5×50 mg
Naloxone	2×1 mg
1 per cent plain lignocaine	5×10 ml

Table 34.2   Flying squad equipment

A delivery pack:
1. Three sterile towels to drape the mother.
2. One sterile towel to wrap the baby.
3. A disposable female urinary catheter.
4. A Galley pot with five cotton wool balls.
5. Savlon antiseptic fluid.
6. Hibitane cream.
7. Episiotomy scissors.
8. Cord scissors.
9. Two pairs of Spencer–Wells forceps.
10. Four plastic cord clamps.
11. Two sterile surgeon's gowns.
12. Two pairs each of sterile gloves from size 5.5 to size 8.5 in 0.5 steps.
13. A mucus extractor.
14. A plastic bag for the placenta.

A perineal repair set:
1. Two pairs of Spencer–Wells forceps.
2. A pair of needle holders.
3. A pair of toothed forceps.
4. A pair of suture scissors.
5. A large vaginal tampon.
6. Five packs of five small gauze squares.
7. Suture material: 2 × 441 CCG

Obstetric forceps
  A pair of each of the following:
1. Wrigley's forceps.
2. Neville–Barnes forceps.
3. Kjelland's forceps.

Infusion fluid
1. Two 1 ℓ of normal saline.
2. Two 1 ℓ of Hartmann's solution.
3. Two 500 ml Haemaccel.
4. Two giving sets suitable for the administration of blood.

Syringes
1. Three 20 ml.
2. Three 10 ml.
3. Three 5 ml.
4. Five 2 ml.

Needles
1. Five green needles.
2. Five blue needles.

Blood bottles
1. Two pink bottles for haemoglobin.
2. Two plain tubes for group and cross-match blood.

Table 34.3   Equipment for neonatal resuscitation

Two straight bladed laryngoscopes.
Three endotracheal tubes (2.5, 3.0, 3.5 mm).
One endotracheal introducer.
Two neonatal airways.
One resuscitation bag.
Appropriate connections for the above.

Two mucus extractors.

This can be performed using a combination of iv pethidine (50 mg) and Entonox for analgesia.

b.   Imminent delivery. In this case it is better to deliver the patient at home. Transfer to hospital after delivery is not necessary if there are no complications.

c.   If the emergency is over by the time the flying squad arrives.

8.   On return to the hospital:

a.   Make detailed notes of the event including call-out time, time of arrival and departure and treatment.

b.   Replace any used equipment or drugs. Inform the blood bank if the blood was used and have it replaced.

Chapter 35
Stillbirth and Neonatal Death

35.1 INTRODUCTION

When a pregnancy terminates tragically with the loss of the fetus or neonate, particular care and support should be provided for the couple involved. It is a particularly difficult time not only for the couple, but also for the staff, friends and family, who often find difficulty coping with the situation and are unsure of the best approach to the bereaved couple. The magnitude of grief at the loss bears little relationship to the timing at which it has occurred. The couple should be given every opportunity to express their grief, since this is a necessary part of a normal recovery process. They will commonly pass through the phases of initial denial of what has occurred, followed by a more aggressive attempt to apportion blame, perhaps on themselves or on hospital staff. This is then followed by eventual acceptance of their loss, which usually takes several months.

Everyone involved with the couple should given them the opportunity to talk about their feelings, and should be alert to the possibility of a pathological grief reaction, which may have serious psychological consequences for the future. This can be recognized by an inappropriate affect, or signs of withdrawal and severe depression. Psychiatric referral should be considered if there are signs of a depressive illness, particularly if suicide is a possibility.

The most appropriate place to nurse a woman who has suffered a stillbirth or neonatal death is probably in a single room on the maternity unit. Although the sight and sound of other healthy babies may be upsetting initially, it is important that she should not feel that she is being isolated, and that midwifery and medical staff should continue to be involved with her.

35.2   DEFINITIONS

35.2.1   Intra-uterine death (IUD)

An IUD refers to the death of the fetus before the onset of labour at any gestation. (The term is usually applied after the first trimester.)

35.2.2   Stillbirth

A stillbirth is defined as the delivery of a dead baby after 28 weeks' gestation. Prior to 28 weeks it is legally termed an abortion, but this term may be upsetting to the patient if she hears it used.

35.3   PROBLEMS ASSOCIATED WITH IUD

1. DIC. About 30 per cent of patients exhibit DIC 3–4 weeks after the IUD has occurred (see Chapter 14).
2. Intra-uterine infection.
3. Induction of labour may be difficult.
4. Psychological and psychiatric sequelae.

35.4   MANAGEMENT OF LABOUR

Once an IUD has been diagnosed, most women do not want to await the onset of spontaneous labour, which may take several weeks. During this time, complications may occur and so it is usually preferable to admit them to the labour ward for induction of labour within a few days, according to their wishes. Care of the patient during labour requires particular sympathy and understanding and ideally should be undertaken by staff already known to the patient. Her partner and/or companions should be encouraged to stay with her at all times. Before her admission, care should be taken to remove fetal heart monitors and related equipment from the room, the sight of which may cause distress.

35.4.1   Investigations

1. Hb.
2. Save serum.
3. Clotting screen (see Chapter 14).

35.4.2   Induction and augmentation of labour

The following guidelines are suggested:
1. Give 3 mg PGE_2 vaginal pessaries 3 hourly until labour commences or until the cervix is ripe enough to accept a 30 FG Foley catheter for an extra-amniotic PGE_2 infusion.
2. If labour commences following PGE_2 pessaries augment with syntocinon according to the usual regimen (see Section 7.3.3).
3. If labour does not occur, start an extra-amniotic infusion of PGE_2 using a syringe pump. Augment with syntocinon if necessary.
4. Do *not* rupture the membranes until the cervix is more than 6 cm dilated.
5. Keep an accurate fluid balance chart.

35.4.3   Analgesia

Analgesia should be given liberally, but sedation should not be excessive because it is important not to suppress emotion which is part of the normal grief reaction.

Opiates, such as morphine or diamorphine can be given as necessary (every 2–3 h) or if the patient wishes she may have an epidural block providing there is no coagulopathy.

35.4.4   Rupture of the membranes

This may be deferred until the patient is well advanced in labour (more than 6 cm cervical dilatation) because of the risks of intra-uterine infection if it is performed too early.

35.4.5   The delivery

If the dead fetus is lying transversely delivery should be by Caesarean section (see Chapter 20). If possible an episiotomy should be avoided as this will only prove to be a painful reminder of the woman's loss. Even when told that her fetus has died, a woman often retains an attitude of disbelief until delivery.

This is therefore a time of renewed grief with the realisation that what she has been told is indeed true.

Parents should be encouraged to see and hold their dead baby which will help them to grieve normally, and accept that the baby is dead. After the baby has been washed and appropriately dressed a Polaroid photograph should be taken and offered to the parents so that they have something with which to remember their baby. If they decline, the photograph should be stored in the notes in case they change their minds in the future. If the baby is expected to be macerated or abnormal it should be explained to the parents and if possible it should be wrapped in such a way that the normal parts of the baby are emphasised and shown to the parents first.

It is important that the parents should not feel rushed, and should be allowed as long as they wish with the baby.

35.5 POSTNATAL CARE

Ideally the woman should continue to be looked after by staff already known to her on the postnatal (or antenatal) ward. Facilities should be available for her partner to stay with her at all times if he wishes. She may not wish to stay long in hospital and as soon as she is medically fit, she should be allowed home. It is of particular importance to ensure that community services and the general practitioner have been informed of the outcome of the pregnancy so that appropriate support will continue to be provided at home.

1. The woman should be asked if she wishes to see the hospital chaplain.
2. Before leaving hospital the parents should be interviewed by the consultant (or his/her deputy) who will explain as far as possible the circumstances surrounding the death.
3. An appointment will be made to see the consultant again in four weeks in a gynaecological out-patients' department or his/her office. The woman should not be brought back to a postnatal clinic.
4. The patient should be given the name and address of the Stillbirth and Neonatal Death Society (see Appendix IV). It should be explained to the parents that the people involved in this association are those who themselves have experienced a perinatal death and who will visit the couple to talk to them if they wish.
5. Lactation can usually be suppressed by means of a firm, supporting brassiere. The woman should be asked to avoid handling the breasts, e.g. after washing she should pat them dry. If necessary 2.5 mg of bromocriptine may be given orally b.d. for 14 days but it may cause nausea.
6. Women who have not only lost their infant but who also needed a *hysterectomy* or women who have *one surviving twin* usually need professional psychotherapeutic help. It is better if this is arranged for them before they leave hospital.
7. It is mandatory that the SHO responsible for the woman must telephone the general practitioner on the day of death so that he/she is aware that the baby has died, and will be able to visit the couple after discharge from hospital.
8. The postnatal ward sister must also inform the health visitor and the community midwife.
9. A check list has been devised by the Royal College of Obstetricians and Gynaecologists (see Table 35.1) which lists items relating to perinatal loss. This can be attached to the patient's notes, and should become the responsibility of one member of staff to ensure that all items on the list have been dealt with.

Table 35.1   Checklist following a stillbirth or neonatal death

Name	Sign and date
Mother informed of death by	
Father informed of death by	
Parents given opportunity to handle baby	
Consultant obstetrician informed	
Consultant paediatrician informed	
Consent for *post mortem* request given/refused (delete)	
Post mortem form completed	
Date and time of *post mortem*	
Date and time of *post mortem*	
Preliminary *post mortem* results explained to mother and father	
General practitioner informed	
Death or stillbirth certificate completed and given to parents	
Informed re. funeral arrangements	
Parents offered booklet 'Loss of your baby'	
Mother seen by social worker Father seen by social worker	
Mother seen by consultant obstetrician Father seen by consultant obstetrician	
Mother seen by consultant paediatrician Father seen by consultant paediactrician	
Religious adviser notified (if desired by patient)	
Chapel service requested/not requested (delete)	
Community midwives notified and/or health visitor	
Postnatal visit date. Clinic Sister notified	
Informed of book of remembrance	
Follow-up visit or phone call	
Photograph taken yes/no Photograph given to parents or kept in case notes	
Case sheet specially marked	

35.6 CONSENT FOR *POST MORTEM*

At an appropriate interval after delivery, it should be explained to every woman who loses her baby that a *post mortem* examination is advisable to attempt to identify the cause of the perinatal death. This will enable the couple to be counselled as to the likelihood of recurrence in the next pregnancy. The duty obstetric registrar should attempt to obtain this permission if the infant is stillborn; in the case of a neonatal death consent is usually obtained by a member of the paediatric team. The parents should be allowed the opportunity to see the baby again, before the *post mortem* is commenced.

If permission is obtained it should be in writing. Having obtained permission an immediate summary of the case should be written on the appropriate *post mortem* request form.

If patients refuse *post mortem* (which is often for religious reasons) the following procedure should be undertaken:

1. Heart blood should be collected for viral studies and karyotyping (see Appendix III).
2. Two Polaroid photographs of the baby should be taken. One should be a general photograph and the other should be a close up (at not less than 3 ft distance) of the baby's face.
3. The baby should be X-rayed as soon as is convenient.

In general points 2 and 3 should be carried out in the *post mortem* room. If possible the hospital photographer should also be asked to photograph the baby as the quality of Polaroids is often poor.

35.7 CERTIFICATION AND INFORMATION FOR THE FATHER

1. If the baby was stillborn a stillbirth certificate should be signed by the SHO or registrar as soon as possible and given to the parents. A fetus that is born without

---

Date

To whom it may concern

This is to certify that I was present at the birth of the baby of .... (enter parent(s) name(s)) who was born before 28 weeks gestation and without signs of life. I should be grateful for your help in arranging for the baby to be buried.

Signed: ....

Qualifications: ....

Position: ....

Figure 35.1 Specimen letter to the undertaker

signs of life before 28 completed weeks gestation is legally an abortion and does not require a certificate. Many patients who lose their babies before 28 weeks wish to bury them and in these cases funeral directors request a certificate from a medical attendant who witnessed the delivery. It should state in writing that the fetus was born with no signs of life (see Figure 35.1). It is important to inform the histopathology department of the parent's wish to bury the baby, as they may then be able to limit their dissection so as to disfigure the body as little as possible.

2. The baby must be examined by a doctor either at the time of delivery or shortly afterwards. The doctor should also examine the placenta and record his/her findings in the notes.

35.8 NURSING PROCEDURE FOR A STILLBIRTH

1. Offer the woman the choice of having the baby washed and dressed in the room or elsewhere.
2. The baby should be weighed and its length and head circumference should be measured and recorded.
3. The baby should be washed and then dressed in an ordinary nightdress and left with the parents as long as they wish. It is important to allow the couple time to be alone to grieve their loss.
4. When the couple no longer wish to see the baby, the baby is dressed in the shroud and disposable nappy.
5. A baby label should be attached to the shroud.
6. A copy of form 151 (death notice) should be attached to the shroud.
7. A copy of the *post mortem* consent form should be attached to the shroud, if the parents have consented.
8. The baby is taken to the mortuary. The porter will use a special box which is used only for this purpose.
9. Three 'death notice' labels are required to be completed by the nursing staff. Ensure one is placed on the baby, one is given to the porter and one is sent to the property office together with the stillbirth certificate.
10. The father of the baby should be instructed to take the stillbirth certificate to the Registrar of Births and Deaths who will issue a certificate of disposal when the death is registered. This certificate is required by the undertaker for the funeral to take place. The father should then take the certificate of disposal to the property office where funeral arrangements will be discussed with administration.

Chapter 36

Destructive Procedures

36.1   Introduction
36.2   Management of a hydrocephalic fetus

36.1   INTRODUCTION

Apart from decompression of a hydrocephalic fetus destructive operations have *no* part to play in obstetric practice in developed countries. This is because the risk of uterine rupture is high and delivery by Caesarean section, even classical Caesarean section, is safer in the hands of most obstetricians.

36.2   MANAGEMENT OF A HYDROCEPHALIC FETUS

1. If a fetus is recognized as being hydrocephalic in late pregnancy an ultrasound assessment should be made to determine the severity of the hydrocephaly and to look for associated lesions, in particular spina bifida.
2. The situation should then be discussed with the parents who should be informed of the likely prognosis based on the ultrasound findings. A Caesarean section is indicated for any of the following reasons:
    a. The parents wish it, having been fully informed of the prognosis.
    b. There is doubt about the severity of the lesion.
    c. The lesion is compatible with a reasonably normal life style.
    Many of these decisions are value judgements and should be made only after consultation with neonatal paediatricians and a paediatric surgeon.
3. If Caesarean section is not justified because the parents do not wish it, the prognosis is grave or the condition is not compatible with viability then the fetal biparietal diameter (BPD) should be measured. In many cases this will be within normal limits. The term hydrocephaly is a misnomer as the fetal head size is often normal even in late pregnancy and it is the cerebral ventricles which are distended. The following guidelines are offered:
    a. If the BPD is normal but the prognosis for the fetus is poor, prolonging the second stage is likely to result in a stillbirth. This obviates the need for perforation operations so avoiding the risk of maternal injury. If the parents

wish the child to be baptised it can usually be arranged for the fetus to be born with a very slow heart rate.

b. If the BPD is too large to permit vaginal delivery then a perforation must be performed. Labour should be induced when the cervix is ripe and adequate analgesia should be provided. At about 5–6 cm of cervical dilatation the scalp over the anterior fontanelle is incised with a scalpel and then a pair of Spencer–Wells forceps is inserted into the fetal brain and directed towards the posterior fossa. The forceps are used to destroy the contents of the posterior fossa until an assistant observes cardiac standstill on a portable real-time machine, with the screen out of the parents' line of vision. At full dilatation delivery is usually completed by means of obstetric forceps.

c. If the BPD is large and the presentation is breech the fetal head may be decompressed either by inserting a metal cannula through the accompanying spina bifida or by incising the skin over the fetal neck and then inserting the Spencer–Wells forceps into the cysterna magna. In the former case the infant way well be born alive whereas in the latter the contents of the posterior fossa may be destroyed as described above.

Chapter 37

Legal Aspects of Labour and Delivery

37.1   INTRODUCTION

Patients are now becoming more litigation-conscious and this, combined with a demand for greater consumer choice in the management of labour and delivery, often puts the obstetrician in a difficult position. This chapter attempts to give some guidelines as to how to manage the more commonly encountered situations. It is by no means comprehensive and in difficult or worrying situations the advice of the Medical Defence Union or Medical Protection Society should be sought.

37.2   BIRTH PLANS

It is now increasingly common for a pregnant woman to provide her midwife or obstetrician with an outline of the way in which she would like her labour to be managed. Ideally these plans will be discussed in detail during an antenatal visit between the woman, her partner and the midwife and consultant. The following guidelines may help:

1. Do not be hostile towards the woman's requests. If time does not permit a full discussion organize another appointment. It is vital that birth plans are discussed fully antenatally to avoid controversy in labour.
2. Discuss each part of the requests in detail, attempting to discover why the request has been made and then interpret it in the light of the facilities and staff available in your hospital. If this is done many misunderstandings are often cleared up.
3. Be reasonable in your personal views. For instance there is little scientific evidence that routine continuous electronic intrapartum FHR monitoring of low risk pregnancies is justified. This is especially so for women belonging to higher social classes. Most patients will agree to intermittent external monitoring (see Section 2.2) and will accept full monitoring, after explanation, if a problem arises in labour.
4. Do not make unrealistic promises. It is unwise to promise a woman an epidural on demand if you do not have anaesthetists whose sole responsibilities are on the labour ward for 24 h each day.
5. Organize regular trips around your labour ward so that local facilities (or lack of them) are appreciated by the women.
6. Hold regular policy meetings with labour ward staff so that a sympathetic attitude towards labour can be encouraged.
7. Encourage partners, relatives and physiotherapists or National Childbirth Trust teachers to be present throughout labour and delivery.
8. If you have strong views on aspects of the management of labour and you cannot persuade the patient to accept them the following choices are available:
   a. Transfer the patient to a colleague who has sympathetic views.
   b. Refer the patient back to her general practitioner with a request for her to be booked urgently at another hospital.
   c. If either of these is impossible and both you and the woman feel strongly then ask her to sign a disclaimer in the notes. This is a last resort as it invariably causes intense hostility.
9. Record the conversation and the essence of the agreed deviations from standard labour ward protocol in the woman's notes so that they are available to the labour ward staff when she is admitted. If the patient offers a written birth plan file it in the notes with your comments.
10. Finally when the woman is in labour attempt to explain your proposed line of action and get her verbal consent before performing any manoeuvre.

37.3   CAN WOMEN DEMAND A LINE OF MANAGEMENT?

This is not a common situation but may produce more problems than birth plans. The most commonly encountered demands during time of labour are:

1. Request for induction for social reasons. If the cervix if favourable (Bishop's score of more than six) and the social reason is pressing most obstetricians will agree to the patient's request after having duly recorded it in the notes. If the cervix is not favourable and induction is likely to fail this should be put to the patient. If she is still insistent a value judgement has to be made but having fully explained the risks of a failed induction many obstetricians will agree to the patient's wishes.
2. A request for Caesarean section. This usually comes from a patient who either had

a prolonged first labour that ended as a Caesarean section or who had a damaged baby following vaginal delivery. In both of these circumstances it is very reasonable to acquiesce to the patient's wishes having recorded the reasons in the notes. Occasionally women ask for a Caesarean section because of an unfounded fear. For instance if a woman has had genital herpes she may be aware of the poor prognosis from neonatal systemic herpes infections. Usually a detailed explanation and the offer of cervical swabs for herpes culture at fortnightly intervals from 36 weeks of gestation will reassure the woman.

37.4   JEHOVAH'S WITNESSES

These women will usually refuse a blood transfusion even if it means that they will die. Many doctors are not prepared to stand and watch a patient die for want of a blood transfusion. If a Jehovah's witness offers herself as a patient her views on transfusion should be sought. The worst possible situation arises when both parties hope that the occasion will never arise and then a transfusion becomes necessary. The following guidelines may help:

1. Some Jehovah's witnesses wish to avoid transfusion except where it is a matter of life and death. This is a situation that most doctors can accept.
2. Those Jehovah's witnesses who will not accept a transfusion under any circumstances can be asked to sign a disclaimer absolving the doctor and the health authority from blame in the case of death from refusal.
3. If you cannot accept point 2 it is preferable to arrange to transfer the patient to the care of another consultant.
4. If you do not look after strict Jehovah's witnesses and you encounter one in an emergency situation you must act as your conscience dictates. If you transfuse the patient who has expressly withheld her permission, for instance whilst she is under general anaesthetic she would legally be entitled to sue. The outcome of such a case is not known as it has never happened to the best of our knowledge.

37.5   CONSENT

Consent in medicine is of three types:

1. Implied. For example, the presence of the woman in the clinic implies their consent to examination (excluding rectal and/or vaginal examinations).
2. Verbal. This is usually requested before rectal or vaginal examinations and prior to such procedures such as ARM or episiotomy.
3. Written. This is required before all operations, but may be omitted in cases of genuine emergency or when the patient is unable to consent (e.g. she is unconscious).

37.5.1   Age of consent

In Great Britain the legal age of consent is sixteen years. Below this age a parent or guardian's signature is required. It is wise, therefore to encourage a parent to stay with a woman of less than sixteen years of age whilst she is in labour. In an emergency it may be overlooked.

37.5.2   Consent for epidural

This must be obtained in writing by the anaesthetist (or obstetrician) who is to carry out the procedure.

37.5.3   Consent for operative deliveries

As a general rule verbal consent is obtained for forceps deliveries, assisted breech deliveries and Ventouse extractions but written consent should be obtained for Caesarean section. Written consent is only valid if a reasonable explanation of the reasons, the procedure and its complications have been given. If the situation is urgent, for example, following a cord prolapse or an abruption, verbal consent will suffice but the reason for the absence of written consent should be recorded in the notes after delivery.

37.5.4   Consent by spouse

This is usually requested when the patient is unable to sign her own consent because:
1. She is mentally incapable, e.g. she is heavily sedated or mentally retarded.
2. She is physically unable to do so, usually because of multiple intravenous lines.
3. It is usual for the husband to consent. This is commonly the case with Arabic wives and women from Bangladesh.

37.5.5   Consent for sterilization

Consent for sterilization should be obtained antenatally and preferably in the first half of pregnancy. Although the law requires only the signature of the person undergoing the operation it is wisest to see both partners, discuss the implications and then to obtain both signatures on a specially designed form. The procedure, its aim, its failure rate and its complications must be explained.

Sterilization carried out at the time of Caesarean section or in the immediate puerperium has the following additional complications:

1. It is performed when the baby is only minutes or hours old. The risks of dying in the perinatal period are greater than dying as an infant.
2. It has double the failure rate of non-pregnancy related procedures, approximately six to eight failures per 1000 women sterilized.
3. It increases the risk of puerperal thromboembolism.

It is preferable therefore to delay the procedure by six weeks. Alternative contraception, possibly Depot Provera should be offered.

Consent for sterilization obtained in labour is not valid.

Appendix I

List of High Risk Factors Indicating Need for Assessment of the Woman in Labour by the Duty Registrar

I.1 FACTORS PRESENTING BEFORE LABOUR

1. Primigravidae aged 35 or over.
2. Multigravidae aged 40 or over.
3. Grand-multiparae (that is more than four deliveries after 28 weeks gestation).
4. Poor obstetric history (previous stillbirth, neonatal death or multiple miscarriages).
5. Previous uterine scar.
6. Any major medical complication.
7. Rhesus iso-immunization.
8. Any woman with a blood pressure of 140/90 mmHg or more.
9. Antepartum haemorrhage.
10. Multiple pregnancy.
11. Threatened or established preterm labour (before 37 weeks).
12. Known or suspected fetal growth retardation.
13. Abnormal or doubtful presentation or lie.
14. High fetal head at onset of labour.
15. Known fetal abnormality.

I.2 FACTORS PRESENTING DURING LABOUR

1. Unbooked women or those who have received no antenatal care.
2. A breech presentation or other malpresentation diagnosed in labour.
3. Meconium staining of the amniotic fluid.
4. Supine hypotension.
5. Pyrexia (that is any woman with a temperature of more than 37.5 °C).
6. Hypertension (that is a blood pressure of more than or equal to 140/90 mmHg).
7. Dysfunctional labour (that is any woman who falls 2 h (or more) to the right of Studd's nomogram of cervical dilatation (see Section 8.2).
8. Abnormal fetal heart pattern on CTG.
9. Prolonged second stage.

Appendix II

Indications for Calling a Paediatrician to be Present at Delivery

1. Preterm babies (less than 37 weeks completed gestation).
2. Fetal distress, diagnosed either by an abnormality of the fetal heart rate or by an abnormal scalp pH.
3. Meconium staining of the amniotic fluid.
4. Prolonged rupture of the membranes (over 24 h).
5. Maternal pyrexia.
6. Intra-uterine growth retardation.
7. Multiple pregnancy. There should be a paediatrician present for each baby.
8. Operative delivery including breech delivery, all Caesarean sections and any delivery requiring general anaesthesia for the mother. It is not necessary to have a paediatrician present at low forceps delivery, unless there has been fetal distress.
9. Known or suspected fetal abnormality.
10. Rhesus iso-immunization.
11. Maternal diabetes mellitus.
12. Maternal hypertension of sufficient degree to warrant drug therapy.
13. Severe antepartum haemorrhage.
14. Shoulder dystocia.

Appendix III

Indications for Taking Cord Blood at Delivery

Indications are given in Table III.1.

Table III.1   Indications for taking cord blood at delivery

Indication	Requirements	Amount
Rhesus negative mothers	Pink tube[a]	5 ml
	White tube[b]	10 ml
Other atypical antibodies	Pink tube[a]	5 ml
	White tube[b]	10 ml
History of:		
Positive syphilis serology	White tube[b]	10 ml
Positive Australia antigen	White tube[b]	10 ml
Rubella in pregnancy	White tube[b]	10 ml
Sickle cell trait/disease	Pink tube[a]	5 ml
Stillbirth	White tube[b] (for torch screen)	10 ml
	Orange tube[c] (for chromosomes)	5 ml
Suspected twin–twin transfusion	Pink tube[a]	5 ml from each cord
Blood gases	(see below)	

[a] Pink tube (EDTA as anticoagulant)
[b] White tube (no anticoagulant)
[c] Orange tube (lithium heparin as anticoagulant)

III.1   METHOD

Clean the proposed site with a Mediswab. Obtain the blood from the cord or a large placental vessel by means of a needle and syringe. It *must not* be squeezed out of the end of the cord as it will be contaminated. This is especially true for Australia antigen positive patients.

III.2   BLOOD GASES

Ideally all deliveries should have a blood gas performed on the blood obtained from the umbilical vein. If this is not possible it should at least be attempted on all operative deliveries and in all cases of fetal distress.

III.2.1   Method

1. After clamping and cutting the umbilical cord put a further pair of Spencer–Wells forceps about 20 cm (8 in) along the cord in the direction of the placenta.
2. After delivery of the placenta take 2 ml of blood into a previously heparinized syringe from the portion of the cord between the two clamps. Mix the blood and heparin well.
3. Expel any air from the syringe. If blood gas analysis is not done immediately cap the syringe.

Appendix IV
Useful Addresses

1. The Stillbirth and Neonatal Death Society (SANDS)
   Argyle House
   29–31 Euston Road
   London NW1 2SD
   01–833 2851
2. Cleft Lip and Palate Association (CLAPA)
   Dental Department
   Hospital for Sick Children
   Great Ormond Street
   London WC1N 3JH
   01–405 9200 Ext. 316
3. National Association for Spina Bifida and Hydrocephalus
   Tavistock House North
   Tavistock Square
   London WC1H 9HJ
   01-388 1382
4. National Childbirth Trust
   9 Queensborough Terrace
   London W2 3TB
   01-221 3833
5. Twins and Multiples Birth Association
   c/o Katy Gow
   292 Valley Road
   Lillington
   Warwickshire CV32 7UE
6. Sickle Cell Society
   Green Lodge
   Barretts Green Road
   NW10 7AP
   01-961 7795
   01-961 8346

Appendix V
Abbreviations

A

AA	Australia antigen positive patient
AF	atrial fibrillation
ADH	antidiuretic hormone
AIDS	acquired immune deficiency syndrome
APH	antepartum haemorrhage
ARM	artificial rupture of the membranes

B

b.d.	twice a day (twelve hourly)
BP	blood pressure
BV	baseline variability

C

CCG	chromic catgut
CMV	cytomegalovirus
cm	centimetre
CNS	central nervous system
CPD	cephalopelvic disproportion
CTG	cardiotocograph
CVP	central venous pressure

D

DC	direct current
DIC	disseminated intravascular coagulation
dl	decilitre
DVT	deep vein thrombosis

E

ECG	electrocardiograph
EUA	examination under anaesthetic

F

FBS	fetal blood sample
FDPs	fibrin and fibrinogen degradation products
FFP	fresh frozen plasma
FG	French gauge
FHR	fetal heart rate
FHRM	fetal heart rate monitor(ing)
FSE	fetal scalp electrode

G

g	gram(s)

H

h	hours
Hb	haemoglobin
HB_eAb	hepatitis B e antibody
HB_eAg	hepatitis B e antigen
HB_sAg	hepatitis B surface antigen
Hg	mercury
HIV	human immunodeficiency virus
HOCM	hypertrophic obstructive cardiomyopathy
HTLV3	human T-lymphocyte virus 3
HVS	high vaginal swab

I

i.m.	intramuscular
i.u.	international units
IUC	intra-uterine catheter
IUCD	intra-uterine contraceptive device
IUD	intra-uterine death
IUGR	intra-uterine growth retardation
i.v.	intravenous
IVH	intraventricular haemorrhage

J

JVP	jugular venous pressure

K

KCl	potassium chloride
kPa	kiloPascal

L

ℓ	litre
LFTs	liver function tests
LMA	left mento–anterior
LMP	left mento–posterior
LMT	left mento–transverse
L/S	lecithin-sphyngomyelin ratio
LSCS	lower segment Caesarean section

M

μg	microgram
mEq	milli equivalent
mg	milligram
min	minute
ml	millilitre
mm	millimetre
mmol	millimole
mu	milliunit
MPA	medroxyprogesterone acetate
MSU	mid-stream specimen of urine

N

NICU	neonatal intensive care unit
NIL	not in labour
NND	neonatal death

O

OA	occipito-anterior
OP	occipito-posterior
OT	occipito-transverse

P

PAWP	pulmonary artery wedge pressure
PDL	primary dysfunctional labour
PE	pulmonary embolism
PGE_2	prostaglandin E_2
$PGF_{2\alpha}$	prostaglandin $F_{2\alpha}$
PLP	prolonged latent phase
PNM	perinatal mortality
PNMR	perinatal mortality rate
POP	progesterone only pill
PPF	plasma protein fraction
PPH	postpartum haemorrhage
PPROM	preterm, premature rupture of the membranes
PROM	premature rupture of the membranes
PTG	phosphatidylglycerol

Q

q.d.s.	four times a day (six hourly)

R

RDS	respiratory distress syndrome

S

SACD	secondary arrest of cervical dilatation
SB	stillbirth
s.c.	subcutaneous
SC	sickle cell disease with haemoglobins S & C
SHF	sponge holding forceps
SHO	senior house officer
SRM	spontaneous rupture of the membranes
SS	sickle cell disease with haemoglobin S only
SThal	sickle cell disease with thalassaemia
SVT	supraventricular tachycardia

T

t.d.s.	three times a day (eight hourly)
TORCH	collective term for toxoplasma, rubella, cytomegalovirus and herpesvirus

U

U + E   urea and electrolytes

V

VE   vaginal examination
VF   ventricular fibrillation
VT   ventricular tachycardia

Further Reading

Coagulation Problems During Pregnancy (1985), Letsky, E.A. Churchill Livingstone, Edinburgh.

Litigation in Obstetrics and Gynaecology (1985), Royal College of Obstetrics and Gynaecology, London.

Medical Disorders in Obstetric Practice (1984), De Swiet, M. (ed.) Blackwell Scientific Publications, Oxford, UK.

Progress in Obstetrics and Gynaecology, Studd J.W.W. (ed.) Volumes 1–6 Churchill Livingstone, Edinburgh.

Obstetrical Ultrasound: How, Why and When (1986), Chudleigh, P., and Pearce, J.M.F. Churchill Livingstone, Edinburgh.

Operative Obstetrics (Munro Kerr's) (1977), Myerscough, P.R. (ed.) 9th edition, Bailliere Tindall, London.

Problems in Obstetric Anaesthesia (1987), Morgan, B. (ed.) John Wiley and Sons, Chichester, UK.

Risks of Labour (1986), Crawford, J.W. (ed.) John Wiley and Sons, Chichester, UK.

The Management of Labour (1985), Studd, J.W.W. (ed.) Blackwell Scientific Publications, Oxford, UK.

The Active Management of Labour (1986), O'Driscoll, K., and Meagher, D. Ballière Tindall (UK)

Index